The Teacher Practitioner in Nursing, Midwifery and Health Visiting

Peter Jarvis and
Sheila Gibson

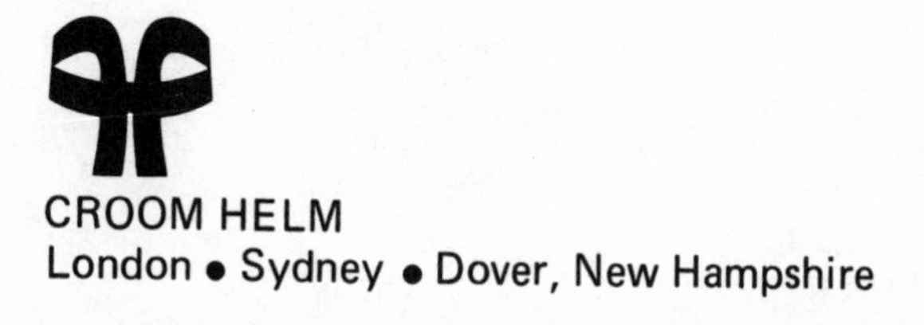

CROOM HELM
London • Sydney • Dover, New Hampshire

Croom Helm Ltd, Provident House, Burrell Row,
Beckenham, Kent, BR3 1AT

Croom Helm Australia Pty Ltd, Suite 4, 6th Floor,
64-76 Kippax Street, Surry Hills, NSW 2010, Australia

Reprinted 1986

British Library Cataloguing in Publication Data

Jarvis, Peter
The teacher practitioner in nursing, midwifery
and health visiting.
1. Medicine—Study and Teaching—Great
Britain 2. Professional education—Great
Britain
I. Title II. Gibson, Sheila
610'.7'1141 R772

ISBN 0-7099-1437-7

Croom Helm, 27 South Main Street,
Wolfeboro, New Hampshire 03894-2069, USA

Library of Congress Cataloging in Publication Data

Jarvis, Peter.
Teaching professional practice in nursing, health
visiting, and midwifery.

Bibliography: p.
Includes index.
1. Community health nursing—study and teaching.
2. Home nursing—study and teaching. 3. Obstetrics—
study and teaching. 4. Midwives. I. Gibson, Sheila.
II. Title. (DNLM: 1. Community Health Nursing—
education. 2. Education, nursing. 3. Nurse
midwives—education. 4. Teaching—methods—nurses'
instruction. WY 18 J38T)
RT98.J37 1985 610.73'43'076 85-5950
ISBN 0-7099-1437-7 (pbk.)

Printed and bound in Great Britain by
Biddles Ltd, Guildford and King's Lynn

CONTENTS

List of Figures
List of Tables
Acknowledgements

Introduction 1

Chapter 1 The Roles of the Teacher Practitioner 3

The Professional Clinical Practitioner 4
The Teacher 6
Straddling Two Professionalisms 7
The Teacher Practitioner within Professional Education and Training 9
Conclusion 11

Chapter 2 The Teaching and Learning Transaction 12

The Teacher Learner Relationship 14
Interpersonal Skills 16
The Roles of the Teacher 18
Conclusion 21

Chapter 3 Designing a Learning Programme 22

The Main Elements of the Curriculum 22
The Design of Learning Experiences 31

The Concept of Need 32
The Notion of Diagnosis 33
Implementing and Managing a Learning Programme 34
Conclusion 36

Chapter 4 Adult Learning 38

Theories of Learning 39
The Learning Cycle 41
Adult Learning 44
Cognitive Learning Styles 46
Learning in the Affective Domain 47
Learning Skills 50
Conclusion 51

Chapter 5 Teaching Adults in Individualised Teaching and Learning 53

Relationship between Theory and Practice 54
Teaching Styles and Models of Teaching 57
Teaching Methods for Individualised Teaching and Learning 59
Some Other Teaching Methods 69
Teaching Aids 72
Preparing a Teaching and Learning Session 75
Conclusion 77

Chapter 6 Assessing Students 78

The Nature of Assessment 78
Rationale for Assessment 80
Types of Assessment 81
Techniques in Assessment 83
Peer and Self Assessment 86
Teaching the Art of Self Assessment 87
Conclusion 88

Chapter 7 Perspectives on the Educational Process 90

The Implementation of a Course for Professional Preparation 90
Philosophical Perspectives on the Educational Process 92
Sociological Perspectives on the Educational Process 95
Conclusion 99

Chapter 8 Creating a Role 100

The Expectations of the Role Set 100
Evaluation of Role Performance 101
Conclusion 102

Suggested Further Reading 103

Bibliography 106

Index 114

LIST OF FIGURES

3.1	A Model of the Curriculum - following Giles et al	23
3.2	A Curriculum Model - following Nicholls and Nicholls	24
3.3	Maslow's Hierarchy of Needs	32
4.1	An Experiential Learning Cycle - following Kolb and Fry	42
5.1	A Problem Solving Cycle	56

LIST OF TABLES

2.1	Some Possible Teaching and Learning Situations	13
4.1	Adult Development and Learning	45

ACKNOWLEDGEMENTS

The idea of this book grew out of our involvement in the preparation of district nurses and health visitors for their teacher practitioner role in courses organized at the University of Surrey and we are grateful to them for the opportunities that we have had to crystallize some of our ideas through interaction with them. In addition, we are extremely grateful to Juliet Clark, Sonia Marshall, Kay Thomas and Lorna Wells who, in their various ways, have assisted in the preparation of the camera ready copy of this manuscript.

Peter Jarvis
Sheila Gibson
University of Surrey

INTRODUCTION

Throughout this book the term 'teacher practitioner' is employed to describe a nurse, midwife or health visitor who is a clinical practitioner but who also has a designated role for teaching students of the appropriate discipline. Among the practitioners who have such a role are:

- clinical nurse teachers
- ward sisters, charge nurses and staff nurses
- fieldwork teachers
- practical work teachers
- midwives, either in hospital or the community
- clinical nurse specialists with either a teaching or a supervisory function
- school nurses who supervise students
- other registered nurses whose role has a teaching component

This text has been written for all teacher practitioners: its main aim is to provide information and ideas about teaching and learning in situations where one teacher is involved with one student, or at the most with a small group of learners. Individualised teaching and learning is used throughout this book to refer to the teaching and learning transaction in which one teacher teaches one learner. A theoretical basis is provided here for this much neglected but very important area of professional education; it attempts to draw theory and practice together, so that teacher practitioners may use the ideas contained in these pages in their every day teaching role.

The opening chapter examines the dual role of the teacher practitioner and some of the problems that this complex role creates are analysed. The following chapter seeks to highlight the essence of the teaching and learning transaction, as an interpersonal relationship requiring certain skills. The third, fourth and fifth chapters outline some of the main elements of adult learning and teaching skills in this interpersonal situation. These chapters form the core of this text. Chapter six examines the process of assessment, an area that in the writers' experiences has caused many teacher practitioners a great deal of concern. The penultimate chapter introduces readers to a slightly broader perspective, helping them to examine the educational process in which the teacher practitioner is involved. Finally, the book returns to the role of the teacher practitioner and considers the ways in which she can create and evaluate her own role performance. The book concludes with a list of suggested texts for further reading, a bibliography and an index.

It should be noted that the female gender is used throughout this text to refer to both teacher practitioners and nurse learners although it is appreciated that the male gender would also be appropriate in some instances.

Chapter One

THE ROLES OF THE TEACHER PRACTITIONER

The teacher practitioner is a nurse, midwife or health visitor whose occupational commitment involves her in both the practice of her branch of nursing and in teaching learners about the role. While it might be justifiably claimed that every qualified nurse has this duty, there are certain roles where the duty is particularly specified by reason of the designation and specification of the post. Some of these roles are listed in the Introduction, but taking the description of one of them, as a example:

> Fieldwork teachers are responsible for teaching the practical aspects of health visiting and for demonstrating the skills and attitudes needed by the health visitor within a variety of social and family settings. They provide opportunities for students to exercise, develop and extend their health visiting skills and in conjunction with nurse managers, lecturers in health visiting and other college staff, they assist in the assessment of the student's potential to become a competent health visitor. They are members of the health visiting staff of a health authority but should also be closely associated with the health visitor course and the training institution concerned.
>
> (Rules, Regulations, Notes for Guidance and Syllabuses for Courses, 1982:12)

While fieldwork teachers (health visitors), practical work teachers (district nurses) and clinical nurse teachers undertake special educational training for their role, other clinical practitioners, i.e., ward sisters and midwives, are not expected necessarily to have been trained in their teaching role before they perform it. Their experience as practitioners has until very recently been considered sufficient for them to perform a teaching role. Some of these practitioners have sought training and undertaken such courses as the London Institute of the City and Guilds 730 course in order to help them in their role performance. However, slowly more specific courses are now being developed which relate to the teacher practitioner role.

Thus it may be seen that the teacher practitioner has a dual role: she is both a practitioner and a teacher. But both roles may be full-time in themselves: nursing is certainly full time and so may teaching adults be a full time occupation. This latter point is certainly true in nursing, midwifery and health visiting where a full time teaching role has emerged and its function is to teach learners about the theory underpinning their occupational role and also to help them to acquire a professional self-identity. Yet many of these teachers now find it difficult to make sufficient time to practise their discipline on the wards or in the community, simply because of the demands of their teaching role. Hence, the role for the teacher practitioner is a very significant one, it is at the interface of theory and practice. Yet this teaching role has been strangely neglected by many professions, the learner being treated rather like an apprentice observing the master at work and seeking to emulate his practice when the master has the time to allow him the opportunity. Some branches of nursing have been much more far sighted than this, creating both a role and providing opportunity for some experienced practitioners to be prepared for it. The extent to which the training is adequate remains largely unresearched, but Battle and Salter (1981:20) discovered that the practical work teachers that they interviewed were mainly satisfied with their preparation. However, there is a need for more research into the preparation of teacher practitioners in a variety of situations.

The teacher practitoner's role is not merely an amalgam of the two roles that describe it, it is an important specialist occupation in its own right. The role of the teacher practitioner, consequently constitutes the focus of this opening chapter, whilst subsequent ones develop the educational theory underlying the teaching aspect of the role. Whilst some application of theory is undertaken, it is not possible to apply all the theoretical aspects to each situation in which the teacher practitioner functions. Neither is any attempt made in this short text book to discuss the occupational role specific to the branch of nursing within which the teacher practitioner may function. The remainder of this chapter, is divided into four main sections: the professional clinical practitioner; the teacher; straddling two professionalisms; the teacher practitioner within professional education and training.

I The Professional Clinical Practitioner

The majority of practising hospital and community nurses, midwives and health visitors are practitioners, although it does need to be recognised from the outset that those managers and teachers who no longer actually practise in the clinical situation are non-effective, in this respect, within the occupation. Therefore, the extent to which they should regard themselves as practitioners is a debatable question.

Yet the occupations in which all the aforementioned practise have been much concerned in recent years to claim that they are professions. Many claims have been made, for instance, that nursing is now a profession, e.g., Hall (1973), Hoy and Robbins (1980). But these claims rest on simplistic conceptions of 'profession'. However, it is not the purpose of this section to enter into this debate, since it is one that is rather sterile and unproductive. Suffice it to note that the debate is so complex that some scholars e.g., Vollmer and Mills (1966:vii) suggest that the word 'profession' does not actually correspond to any reality but rather to an ideal type into which various occupations are seeking to change themselves. Since change is endemic and the concept of profession is static, they prefer to use the idea of 'professionalisation' as being one that corresponds much more to the reality of change.

The concern of this section is, however, with the term 'professional' since this is a much more significant and meaningful concept. This term has at least three meanings

- one who receives remuneration for services rendered
- one who is a member of an occupation which regards itself as a professional
- one who is an expert and who utilises that expertise in the service of the client

It is very important to note that even if the first two are true, it does not necessarily mean that the third is true, nor does the validity of the third imply that the other two must be true as well. But it is the third meaning that constitutes the basis of this section: the professional is one who is an expert and who uses that expertise for the benefit of the client.

But, it might be asked, who is the client of the teacher practitioner? Clearly there are two sets of clients for the teacher practitioner: the patients/clients and the learners. Hence, the expertise referred to in this case is a dual expertise of both the practice of the occupation and the ability to teach it. Before the implications of this point are developed, it is necessary to understand the significance of this meaning of the term to any form of practice.

It follows from the idea that the professional is one who has both the knowledge and skill to respond competently, and to know that she has done so, in every occupational situation. But knowledge is always changing and new skills are having to be acquired, so that the professional practitioner must ensure that she makes time to learn that new knowledge, by reading books, academic and professional journals, attending academic conferences etc, and also by seeking to acquire and practise the new skills. The professional practitioner is one who keeps abreast with new developments in the theory and practice of her occupation.

Clearly this is a responsiblity that every practitioner has to her clients or patients and, as different branches of nursing professionalise, it is important for the practitioners to continue to master new developments that emerge. Hence, it is claimed here that the level of professionalism of practitioners is a much greater concern than to know whether, or not, an occupation regards itself as a profession.

The teacher practitioner therefore, has a double responsibility. Not only does she have to be a professional clinical practitioner in order to employ her knowledge and skill for the benefit of her patients or clients, but she also uses it in order to assist students to learn about the occupation for which they are being prepared. If her knowledge or skill is deficient not only will the patients or clients be put at risk, students entering the occupation will not have had the best introduction that they might have received, for the teacher practitioner will almost certainly become a role model for her learners. However, it must be recognised that not only has the teacher practitioner the duty to be a professional clinical practitioner in her branch of practice but she should also be a professional teacher.

II The Teacher

Malcolm Knowles (1980:26) claims that many people perform a teaching role and, indeed, they do. However, they do not all have to be teacher trained in order to teach, since anybody who facilitates another's learning may be regarded as an educator. Even so, in the case of the teacher practitioner, the role is much more specific since it involves inducting the student into the work situation, which may be located in a ward, a community setting, in a department in a school or college. Yet it is more than merely a process of induction, it is an active teaching role in an interpersonal situation. Two points arise from this:

- it is the role of an educator of adults
- it is performed in an interpersonal situation

There is an increasingly significant body of knowledge emerging about the art of teaching adults and some research results are beginning to appear about individualised learning, so that it is important for the teacher practitioner to be aware of this work. Unfortunately, little has yet been published about the art and science of teaching adults in an interpersonal, one-to-one situation.

However, it may be seen that the practice of teaching adults should be based upon a body of knowledge, in the same way as in the professional practice discussed earlier.Indeed, similar debates have occurred within teaching about the extent to which teaching is a profession, as have arisen within nursing. These discussions are equally sterile, since it is not really of consequence whether or not teaching is a profession, but it is important that teachers should be professionals. Hence, it is much more significant to enquire whether the teacher practitioner is a professional teacher than to ask whether she is a member of two professions. The teacher practitioner should be an expert in teaching adults in an interpersonal situation; she should have both the knowledge and skill to undertake this role with competence. Additionally, since the body of knowledge in the education of adults is expanding rapidly, she should be endeavouring to keep abreast with all of these developments, so that she can offer her learners the most expert service. Hence, the teacher practitioner should be both a professional teacher and a professional practitioner in order to perform her role: this combination of professionalisms is the essence of her occupational role.

III Straddling Two Professionalisms

The teacher practitioner is, therefore, in a most interesting position, she straddles two professionalisms and should be an expert in both. Such a role has its own responsiblities, rewards and problems. As previously mentioned, the teacher practitioner is expected to keep abreast with new knowledge and skills in her practice but at the same time she is required to be aware of new educational knowledge and to be skilful in the manner in which she facilitates the learning of her students. But there is only a limited amount of time for reading and studying and few people are prepared or are able to devote all their leisure to work preparation, so that she is frequently confronted with a dilemma - wherein is she to place her energies? This problem is exacerbated when the teacher practitioner has a heavy workload, since she is still expected to continue her clincial practice as well as to teach the learners. In the ward situation it is possible for the clincial nurse teacher to assume more of the teaching role, so that the ward sister can concentrate on other aspects of her multifaceted role. But this type of co-operation cannot occur in the community where, for instance, the fieldwork teacher and the practical work teacher are independent professional practitioners. Students may, therefore, by viewed as an additional burden to an already overloaded practice. According to the regulations and guidelines governing district nurse education and training a 'practical work teacher should have a reduced but well balanced workload whilst training students.' (Regulations and Guidelines 1983: 13 para 2.10). But it might be equally valid for the practical work teacher to have an increased workload, with additional support staff, so that she can provide a wider and more varied professional practice experience for her student. The same could equally apply to other teacher practitioners working in the community.

Straddling two professional roles has, however, a great many rewards as well as additional responsibilities: it can, for instance, result in job satisfaction at two levels, that of caring for the patient/client and that of helping the student to improve her own practice. This latter aspect has the additional bonus of knowing that the teacher practitioner's own standards of role performance can be maintained and perpetuated, in part, by the way she assists in the preparation of the learner who works with her. Yet it must be recognised that however rewarding the work, straddling two professional roles is both a difficult and demanding task for those who undertake it and it is one that teacher practitioners will inevitably perform in different ways.

Some teacher practitioners may discover that they orientate themselves in the direction of professional practice and get more satisfaction from its performance, others may find more pleasure from performing their teaching role and assisting learners to become more competent practitioners, while a third group may gain satisfaction from both teaching and practising and endeavour to combine both. Given the choice, some teacher practitioners might refuse to take students because their preference is for professional practice. Many others e.g., ward sisters, have little choice and are required to perform both of these roles, plus that of ward manager. However, if clinical nurse teachers and occasionally nurse teachers are available they may be able to assist ward sisters by assuming the teaching role, but this may be the role from which the ward sister gains the most satisfaction. Hence, the clinical nurse teacher does not help the ward sister resolve her dilemma. The clinical nurse teacher's dilemma may not be quite so clear, since she is expected to perform a teaching role in the clinical situation: her dilemma maybe whether she should remain teaching on the wards where she has little influence and control over the students' learning environment since she is not responsible for the overall management of the ward or whether she should spend more time in the school of nursing, which may be expected of her, in order to influence the students' standards and help them to see the relevance of theory to practice.

The teacher practitioner's role straddles two entirely different professionalisms, yet it is a specific role and occupation. It is, in many ways, amongst the most significant in any occupation since it combines theory, practice and the teaching of practice. Nursing, unlike many professions, has begun to recognise the importance of the role and has begun to design educational programmes of preparation for its teacher practitioners, so that the element of practical experience during professional preparation should not degenerate into the expert passing on tips to the learner when she has time, as has been the case in some occupations in the past. The teacher practitioner's role is not only highly skilled but one that requires preparation and it is also very significant because it lies at the interfaces of theory and practice and occupational preparation and practice.

IV The Teacher Practitioner within Professional Education and Training

In students' minds it is easy for theory and practice to become divorced: it is quite common to hear learners, returning to a school or college after a period of professional practical experience, exclaim how much they had enjoyed their practice but how irrelevant the theoretical knowledge appears. A variety of reasons may exist for this, including:

- theory tends to be abstract, generalised and impersonal whereas practice appears concrete, specific and personal
- theory is sometimes taught in an uninteresting fashion and not applied to the actual occupational experience
- the teacher of theory may be far removed from practice and theory may have interest and significance in its own right to the teacher
- modular systems of training may not be in operation and the theory may not be immediately applicable to the students' current work situation

None of these reasons is an excuse for poor teaching but they are offered as examples of reasons why students may feel that the two are so far apart.

Yet a great deal of curriculum knowledge i.e., theoretical knowledge included in the curriculum by the profession's ruling bodies, actually arises from practice and, frequently, knowledge in practice often precedes theoretical generalisation about it. Much of the body of theoretical knowledge (especially that knowledge about how to perform in practice) has emerged from practice and since it has arisen from practice there should be no divorce between it and theory. However, it is here, at the interface of theory and practice, that the teacher practitioner's role is located. The role is to be discovered in the overlap between preparation for practice and practice itself. When the learner takes the initial steps in professional practice, the teacher practitioner guides her in the application of theory to practice and she also assists the learner in drawing out the theoretical implications from the practical experience.

Theoretical knowledge has gained higher status than practical knowledge and so the teacher of theoretical knowledge usually has a more exalted position in the professional hierarchy than has the teacher practitioner. Teaching theory has usually been equated with 'education' while the teaching of practical skills has usually been called 'training'. Education has been regarded as a high status process and training as low status. However, it has been argued elsewhere (Jarvis 1983a) that this distinction is over-simplistic and that training may also be educational. Indeed, in professional education the two should be combined since, while theoretically 'knowledge that' and 'knowledge how' can be separated, professional practice is not a mindless activity. Hence, the preparation of professionals should always be regarded as an educational process, even when they are learning skills. However, there are sociological studies that examine the reasons why theoretical knowledge has high status and practical knowledge has low status e.g., Young (1971), and the fact that this actually occurs does mean that the teacher practitioner, despite her very significant role, usually has lower status than the teacher of theory. She is, therefore, expected to fit her teaching into the demands of the structure of the curriculum that has been planned by teachers of theoretical knowledge, working within the schools of nursing and colleges of further and higher education, although increasingly teacher practitioners are being included in curriculum development and course planning teams. However, even where this occurs, they are usually in the minority. At the same time, it must be recognised that full-time teachers of theory do have an overview of the whole of the learners' preparation. But it would be quite wrong to expect the teacher practitioner to work in isolation from the teaching centre. Indeed, if this were to occur the gulf between theory and practice would be almost unbridgeable. Hence, it is the duty of the tutors in the teaching centre to liaise with the teacher practitioner to ensure that any separation between theory and practice is minimised during the students' preparation and that the whole programme should be regarded as an integrated entity. Only by such liaison can the professional preparation of students become a successful initiation of the learner into professional practice.

The teacher practitioner is at the interface of theory and practice, helping the student to apply theory to practice and to learn from practice and to relate it back to theory. She is, in fact, a key person in the whole educational programme. She can provide an enriching practical experience, stimulating the learner to enjoy the practice of her chosen occupation. However, she has at least two additional roles:

- role model, her role performance might set high standards for her students to emulate

- assessor, since she sees the students perform the professional practice on a continuous basis, so that she is the gate-keeper to the profession

> recommending admittance for those whom she considers have achieved sufficiently high standards but barring others, by use of the current agreed assessment procedures, if she does not consider that they have achieved such standards.

The teacher practitioner therefore, occupies a significant place in the preparation of recruits to the profession: without such a role the education and training of students would be impoverished beyond measure.

Conclusion

This chapter has examined the role of the teacher practitioner, highlighting some of its significant features and illustrating some of its satisfactions and challenges. It is a dual role, practising and teaching, in which there are inherent conflicts and tremendous opportunities. However, the concern of this book is about the teaching element of the role, so that little reference to other features of the role will be made hereafter, until the final chapter, in which a return will be made to the role of teacher practitioner. The next chapter focuses upon the teaching and learning transaction, in which the interaction between the teacher practitioner and the learner is examined.

Chapter Two

THE TEACHING AND LEARNING TRANSACTION

'Transaction' may appear a strange word to employ in this context, since it might be argued that teaching and learning does not involve negotiation because the teacher knows what to teach and the student learns what is taught. This is a very traditional and authoritarian view of education, one that no doubt reflects the experience of many in their initial education and even, perhaps, in their professional preparation. Yet this approach is foreign to the ethos of the education of adults, especially in an individualised teaching and learning situation. Individualised teaching and learning should always be a transaction. Perhaps education itself should always involve negotiation between teacher and learner, even though the status of the teacher in primary education is rather different from that of the five year olds whom she teaches. Education might be defined as 'any planned series of incidents, having a humanistic basis, directed towards the participant(s) learning and understanding.' (Jarvis 1983a:5). This definition presupposes that the humanity of the participant(s) is paramount in the educational process, so that when there is only one teacher and one learner involved it is hardly surprising that some emphasis should be placed upon the interpersonal interaction in the teaching and learning process.

Kidd (1973:269) points out that there are five elements in most teaching and learning transactions.

- the learner
- the teacher
- the group
- the setting or situation
- the subject matter.

In individualised teaching and learning, the group is not present, as Kidd himself recognises. However, there may be occasions when the teacher practitioner has more than one student and while she is instructing one of them, she realises that it would be useful for other learners to join in the learning process, so that she then creates a small group.

The setting, or situation, is a significant element in the transaction in individualised teaching and learning, but it is a feature infrequently mentioned in many textbooks on education because it is automatically assumed that the setting for teaching and learning is the classroom. Some books concerned with the education of adults, e.g. Rogers (1977:101-105), concentrate on the arrangements of furniture in the classroom, suggesting that the desks or tables etc. should be arranged in circles in order to facilitate discussion amongst learners. Yet few writers consider the possibility of either the teacher or the learner choosing the setting in which the transaction might occur. In individualised teaching and learning there may be no classroom teaching, so that the choice of the situation remains with the participants. Often it is the responsibility of the teacher practitioner to decide when the situation is appropriate to raise an issue, but sometimes the learner might wish to question the teacher, so that in this instance it is the learner's responsibility to choose the setting for the transaction to occur. However, when the teacher makes the choice, great care should be given to making a selection in order to ensure that it is most suited for the teaching and learning to occur. The choice may actually involve the teacher practitioner preparing the setting beforehand, but this might not always be necessary, possible or appropriate. Some of the situations in which the teaching and learning transaction might occur are listed overleaf.

Table 2.1: Some Possible Teaching and Learning Situations

For the Ward Sister, Clinical Teacher or Nurse Tutor etc.	For the Fieldwork Teacher, Practical Worker Teacher, Community Teaching Midwife, etc.
Ward/Department	Health Centre Office
Sister's/Charge Nurse's Office	Health Centre Treatment Room
Hospital Corridors	Health Centre Staff Room
Staff Room	House of Client/Patient
Staff Canteen	Car (teacher's or student's)
Seminar/Tutorial Room	Staff Canteen

Clearly some of these locations are rather public and the discretion of the teacher practitioner must be used in all circumstances. It is impolite to teach a student in the presence of the patient/client, unless the latter has agreed that it should happen. In addition, some of the above venues may be rather exposed to other people overhearing the teaching and learning transaction, which might not be appropriate.

Every teacher practitioner is aware of her own work situation, so that she should be cognisant of the possibilities that exist and be prepared to utilise them in an appropriate manner. Some teacher practitioners have been able to negotiate the use of a room in close proximity to their clinical work situation which they can utilise for teaching purposes. This is obviously an ideal situation which enables the teaching and learning to proceed with less disturbance. However, it may be recognised from the above table of venues that the teaching and learning transaction may not always be formalised, ideal, or institutional in nature.

Three other items remain from Kidd's five elements: content will be discussed in the subsequent chapter on designing a learning programme, so that the teacher and the learner elements remain. It is clear from this initial discussion that individualised teaching and learning relies heavily upon human interaction and a prerequisite for its success lies in the establishment of an effective working relationship between the teacher practitioner and the learner. Therefore, the remainder of the chapter explores the teacher-learner relationship, interpersonal skills and some of the different roles of the teacher.

I The Teacher Learner Relationship

The traditional image of the teacher standing before a class of students expounding the mysteries of knowledge about which the teacher is an expert is hardly appropriate to the forms of teaching and learning being discussed here. Neither are the conventional images of the student sitting at the feet of the guru awaiting with patience to receive the pearls of wisdom that he is prepared to cast forth, or of the apprentice looking over the master's shoulder watching the expert at work and thereby hoping to acquire sufficient knowledge to emulate his feats or expertise. Even so, it is recognised that there is a place for the demonstration of skill in the interpersonal teaching and learning situation in which the teacher practitioner participates, but it may not be as significant as some people assume. Nevertheless, this approach is still predominant in some professional spheres but where it occurs it may be regarded as rather anachronistic, reflecting an approach that assumes that teacher practitioners can pass on their skills effectively to the student, simply because they are expert practitioners. Little concern is paid in either of these conventional approaches to the skills of teaching or to the relationship of the teacher with the student. Explicit to this discussion is an emphasis on the inter-personal aspects of the relationship, in which the dignity and humanity of both participants are fully recognised and respected.

Even so, it might be argued that the dignity and the humanity of the participants may still be respected in a hierarchical relationship, with the teacher practitioner exercising the authority of her position over the learner. Radical educators, e.g. Bowles and Gintis (1976), claim that education tends to prepare learners to accept hierarchical relationships in the work situation because teaching and learning is conducted within a hierarchical context. While Bowles and Gintis refer to the school and the education of children, so that the reference may not be totally relevant here, the context in which the education occurs is part of what some scholars regard as the hidden curriculum, a concept that will be discussed below. Nevertheless, it is a social function of education that should not be reproduced in the individualised, nonformal teaching and learning situation within which much of the teacher practitioner's teaching should be conducted. However, it might be realistic to claim that since the majority of learners are going to be employed in the Health Service, which is a fairly rigid hierarchy, they should be prepared within one. Yet the aims of professional education (see Jarvis 1983a:31-49) do not include reproducing the social hierarchy of the employing organisation but rather to produce individuals who can think and act independently and critically in both a work and non-work situation. Hence, the hierarchical approach should be eschewed in individualised teaching and learning, indeed it should seldom be included in any form of education, especially in the education of adults.

Hence, it may be asked, what authority does the teacher practitioner possess, since teacher practitioners usually occupy higher positions in the Health Service hierarchy than do their learners? For instance, the ward sister is responsible for the smooth organisation of the ward and for the standard of nursing care given to the patients within it, while the learners may be accountable to her in part for the care that they render patients. Note, however, that this accountability is for the performance of the nursing role but not for the learning that has occurred in the teaching and learning transaction. The ward sister's authority is that of ward sister rather than that of teacher practitioner. She should gain the respect of her learners because of her knowledge and skill. Similarly, if a fieldwork teacher or a practical work teacher were teaching a senior nurse manager about some technique developed in the community, she would have no authority over the manager, yet she should still command the respect of the senior nurse manager because of her knowledge and skill. The authority of the teacher practitioner is that granted to her by the learner who respects her professionalism. But if she cannot gain that respect, then the teacher practitioner has no authority, as teacher, in the eyes of the learner. Professional authority finds its legitimation in the recognition given to the practitioner by peers, clients and students, but not in the position occupied in the hierarchy. Hence, the authority of the teacher practitioner resides entirely in the recognition of her professionalism.

Yet learners also bring to the teaching and learning transaction their own ideas and experiences, the results of their reading and study, thoughts about new techniques etc. that they have learned in school or college, so that the teacher has also opportunity to learn from the learner. But if there is no genuine relationship as such, interchange might not occur and then the teacher practitioner would not benefit from the student, and as a result she would be intellectually impoverished. It will, no doubt, have been noted that in the definition of education cited earlier in this chapter there was reference to the participants learning but no reference to the teacher. Teachers are not essential to education, but learners are! Teachers are, however, very useful adjuncts to the educational process, but the richer the interchange between teacher and learner and learner and teacher the more both participants are likely to learn. Freire (1972:53) claims that a teacher-student relationship is contrary to the dialogical relationship that should emerge in problem solving learning and he suggests that the relationship should be regarded as a teacher/student - student/teacher one, in which both participants engage in both roles to their mutual benefit.

In individualised teaching and learning, this would appear to be the most appropriate form of relationship that might emerge and the one for which the teacher practitioner should strive. However, it is recognised that this might be difficult to achieve because of the hierarchical environment in which the teaching and learning is transacted, but it is emphasised that its achievement depends upon the skills of the teacher in gaining the co-operation of the learner.

II Interpersonal Skills

It will be apparent from the foregoing discussion that the creation of a relationship of trust and respect is an essential precursor to an enriching teaching and learning transaction. While there is always responsibility on both participants to form such a bond, it must be recognised that the initiative for this lies with the teacher. Hence, it is essential from the outset for the teacher to recognise that her role is not merely that of communicating knowledge and skills to the learner but of creating an environment in which the teaching and learning may be maximised.

Much has been written about interpersonal skills and it would perhaps be unwise to devote too great a space to repeating it here. Nevertheless, it is essential for the teacher practitioner to have self-awareness and to have sufficient self-confidence to step out from behind the barriers of her organisational authority in order to try to create the type of relationship in which the learner can feel free to be herself. This is an extremely difficult undertaking for some people, in the first instance, but the more that the teacher empathises with the learner and seeks to understand the latter's own perception of herself (including her self-confidence and self-esteem), the greater the chance of creating such an environment. In short, the teacher practitioner needs to be both self-confident and sensitive if she is to create a supportive relationship in which the learner has the opportunity to develop as an independent thinker and practitioner.

The teacher should, therefore, spend some time getting to know, on both a personal and a professional level, the student with whom she is working and this may be done before she reads any previous reports about the learner. Student notes are apt to influence the reader and to label the student for the teacher practitioner before the latter sees her perform. It is the responsibility of the teacher practitioner 'to break the ice' with the student in an individualised teaching and learning situation and this may best be done in an informal situation, even away from the work environment if that is possible. Time is always a problem and neither the teacher practitioner nor the learner may have that time, so that an initial meeting may have to occur over a shared coffee break, etc. However, some institutions now try to arrange that the initial informal contact between teacher practitioner and learner is incorporated into the formalised part of the course; this practice is to be encouraged. But wherever it occurs, the first meeting is very important. In a slightly different context, and yet a very similar manner, adult educators recognise the importance of creating the right atmosphere in their class from the outset, so that their preparation for the first meeting may be even more rigorous than that for the classes that they conduct thereafter. The climate created in the first meeting will affect the remainder of the teaching and learning process, so that the teacher practitioner should recognise that the student may:

- be rather anxious and need some reassurance
- have questions about the teaching and learning situation but not the confidence to ask them
- want to know the type of situation in which she will be working, e.g. practice, rules
- want to know some of the expectations that the teacher practitioner has of her
- want to be told about the teaching and learning programme.

Hence, the teacher practitioner should ensure that, from the outset, she invites the student to ask questions and makes certain that adequate time is allowed at their first encounter to answer these in an unhurried and interested manner. Additionally, the teacher may anticipate certain questions and prepare a handout for reference purposes, which she can leave with the student at the end of the first discussion. But during the meeting itself she may merely wish to encourage the learner to talk, ask questions and generally seek to put her at her ease.

Training in interpersonal skills in order to undertake the teacher practitioner role does not always occur in the short courses that are mounted as preparation for this role, even though it may be mentioned in the suggested curriculum. Nevertheless, the teacher practitioner must be aware of the importance of these skills and seek consciously to develop them in her daily work with both her students and her patients/clients. The work environment lends itself to this type of development, since the teacher practitioner is always involved in relationships with her clients, patients, students and peers. The acquisition of the following skills may prove useful for the teacher practitioner, the ability to:

- listen
- hear what is said and note what is left unsaid
- detect emotional signals
- note other non-verbal cues
- respond appropriately in a caring manner.

Teacher practitioners may consider that these are the skills of a sensitive person and ones that should be exercised by any nurse, midwife or health visitor. This is true, since they are the skills upon which the practice of the caring professions are based and it must be recognised that teaching is also a caring profession, so that these skills must be applied quite deliberately in an individualised teaching and learning transaction.

Individualised teaching and learning in a non-formal environment clearly raises questions about the roles that the teacher practitioner performs since it is clear that the teacher is not merely the person who transmits knowledge and skills for the student to acquire.

III The Roles of the Teacher

The role of the teacher practitioner will be discussed in the eighth chapter, but the actual teaching roles in the teaching and learning transaction are discussed here. Once a personal relationship has been established between the teacher and the student, the teacher is exposed to the possibility of playing more parts than just that of the fount of wisdom and the clinical specialist; she may gain the roles of academic adviser and counsellor. While this is not often the teacher practitioner's designated responsibility, since it is quite common for students to have a personal tutor and some colleges also employ the services of a professional counsellor, they are roles that are often played by her and it is difficult not to fulfil these without putting the interpersonal relationship at risk. As academic adviser, the teacher practitioner may be asked by the student: about aspects of the course theory being studied; for help with her course work assignments; about the relationship between theory and practice. As a counsellor, the teacher practitioner may be exposed to some of the problems that the student is experiencing on the course. No teacher practitioner should be expected to be a fully trained counsellor but it is useful to have a minimum of counselling skills to help the student explore the situation so that she can make her own informed decision. She should also have sufficient knowledge to be able to recognise that the problems being experienced by the student are no more than the normal stresses, strains and crises of confidence that students sometimes experience during a course of study or that they are problems that require expert help. However well qualified in counselling the teacher practitioner may be, if she is to concentrate on her teaching role she may wish to refer any student requiring such assistance to the professional student counsellor employed by the school or college, if such a service is available.

The teacher practitioner who establishes a good relationship with the student may well become her 'confidante'. Being entrusted with confidences is a responsibility that the teacher practitioner should expect and respond to in the same manner in which they were shared. Hence, the teacher practitioner should not break any confidence that she is given and if she considers that which she has been told should be revealed to tutors in the college or school of nursing, she should first seek permission from the student to reveal it. Breaking confidence might destroy the relationship that the teacher practitioner has endeavoured to establish and however hard the teacher then tries to re-establish it she will probably not be trusted again by the student, so that it is also doubtful whether she would then be able to fulfil her teaching role effectively.

Not only does the teacher perform these personal roles, she also performs a variety of teaching roles. Kidd (1973:293) suggests that these include:

- animating and inspiring attention and commitment
- presenting information or demonstrating processes(*)
- raising relevant questions, developing habits of self-questioning(*)
- clarifying difficulties or obscurities (*)
- drawing parallels or finding relationships
- reflecting feelings
- expressing agreement and support
- evaluating, or developing the learner's capacity for self-evaluation (*).

Of these eight points the four marked with an asterisk will be developed in detail elsewhere, whilst the remainder are discussed below.

Animating: Most people who embark upon preparation for a profession are highly committed to the idea of entry to that occupation, so that at one level, seeking to inspire commitment is unnecessary. But at another level, in endeavouring to inspire the new entrant to keep abreast with the developments in the theory and practice of the occupation in order to maintain high standards of care, the teacher practitioner may become a role model.

Drawing Parallels and Finding Relationships: Perhaps the most significant element here for the teacher practitioner is in helping the learner to relate theory to practice, so that the divorce between the two does not occur. It is, therefore, essential for the teacher practitoner to know the theory as well as the practice, so that no gulf should appear between the school of nursing or midwifery and the ward, or between the college and the community.

Reflecting Feelings: Practice in any caring profession involves an affective element and the teacher practitioner may have to help the student cope with her emotions at two levels. In the first place, the practice itself may actually involve the learner in having to come to terms with her emotions in caring for her patients/clients and the teacher practitioner should be able to assist in this, e.g. a student health visitor encountering a case of non-accidental injury to a child might feel angry towards the adults who inflicted it, a student nurse encountering death for the first time might feel distraught. In addition, the student may also have an emotional reaction to the learning process that she herself is undergoing, so that the teacher might have to help the student come to terms with this aspect of her professional preparation. The more personal the relationship established between the teacher practitioner and the student the more this role is likely to become apparent. Teachers who are unable to cope with either their own or other people's emotions may be tempted to avoid any form of personal involvement with the student, so that these emotions do not surface in their presence. However, failure to help the student at this level is a failure to perform one of the most important but most neglected aspects of professional preparation.

If the teacher is prepared to acknowledge honestly her own emotions and reactions to stressful situations, especially when these have been previously suppressed, the student may then be willing to do likewise. The mere act of disclosure may create a valuable learning experience where the reasons why professionals react in a variety of ways to difficult encounters can be discussed. In addition, different ways of handling emotions can be considered together.

Expressing Agreement and Support: It is significant that this is specified as a positive rather than a negative response to the learner. Since teacher practitioners are educators of adults they do have to help the learner know when she is correct and when she has made a mistake. However, one of the most stress-inducing responses that a learner can receive is to be told that she is wrong, rather than being helped to reach her own decision that she has made an error and that a specific aspect requires correction. Teachers should always express agreement when the student is correct and always offer support and guidance when she is in error. Praise and support need not always be verbal since non-verbal response may be just as effective. Guidance may not always be in providing the correct answers but in helping the student to think through the problem for herself. This supportive environment is a factor of the teacher-learner relationship that the teacher practitioner should seek to establish since research demonstrates that praise and support produce greater advancement in the learning situation. Reproof, however, has the adverse effect. Carl Rogers (1969) actually concludes that anything but self appraisal may have harmful results.

Each of these roles has been mentioned here because it is an element in the transaction that will not occupy a significant place in the discussion hereafter. Yet each in their own ways are vitally important to the teaching and learning process.

Conclusion

This chapter has begun to explore the teaching and learning transaction in which it is maintained that an open honest dialogue between two human beings is at its heart: both bring themselves, their personalities and their experiences and both learn from each other. Both may share and both may be enriched. One of the privileges of the role of the teacher practitioner is that she can create a supportive environment in which a fellow human being can develop and acquire the knowledge, skills and attitudes appropriate to enter her chosen profession, another is that she may learn as much, or nearly as much, from the person whom she teaches, provided that she succeeds in establishing a relationship in which the learner might also be the teacher.

Having thus explored the teaching and learning transaction, it is now important that elements of student learning should be explored so that the next chapter focuses upon designing learning programmes for students.

Chapter Three

DESIGNING A LEARNING PROGRAMME

The teacher practitioner has two distinct functions in the design of a student's learning experiences: first, as a teacher who performs a role within the broad framework of the curriculum that has been designated by the appropriate professional body and implemented in an approved teaching centre; secondly, as an independent practitioner responsible for designing a learning programme appropriate to the student's learning requirements within the practical experience component of professional preparation. Consequently, the teacher practitioner requires an understanding of the elements of curriculum theory and also some knowledge of the various approaches which can be employed in the design of learning programmes. Therefore, the first two sections of this chapter comprise a discussion of both of these aspects, since they give rise to the significant concept of 'need' and the notion of diagnosis of learning needs, which are considered in the next two sections. The final section elaborates some of the factors involved in implementing and managing a learning programme.

1. The Main Elements of the Curriculum

The term 'curriculum' has a multitude of different meanings so that at the outset of this chapter it is necessary to establish a working definition. Many writers note this confusion of meanings; Kelly (1977:3), for instance, points out that the term is employed to describe a variety of situations from the content of a particular subject or area of study to the total programme of an educational institution. The latter connotation is assumed here and Kerr's (1968:16) definition is adopted, so that the curriculum is taken to be 'all the learning which is planned and guided by the school, whether it is carried on in groups or individually, inside or outside of the school'. Since Kerr's work refers to initial education, as do many of the publications on curriculum, it is necessary to replace the term 'school' with that of 'educational institution'. Hence, the working definition of curriculum adopted here is 'all the learning which is planned and guided by the educational institution, whether it is carried on in groups or individually, inside or outside the institution'. In addition to offering a variety of definitions, curriculum theorists categorize the various elements of the curriculum in different ways. Taba (1962:422) proposed that one way of identifying these elements is to consider the major points at which decisions need to be taken in the process of curriculum development, and suggested that these are:

- aims and objectives
- content
- learning experiences
- evaluation

The majority of curriculum theorists use these elements although 'learning experiences' is often replaced by 'teaching methods' in which both teaching and learning are emphasised, and 'evaluation' is sometimes recognised as including the assessment of learning outcomes while in other schemes it is viewed as a separate entity from assessment.

The interrelationship of these elements of the curriculum has been stressed for a number of years and, for example, Giles, McCutcheon and Zechiel (cited Taba 1962:425) depict it thus:

Figure 3:1 A Model of the Curriculum - following Giles et al

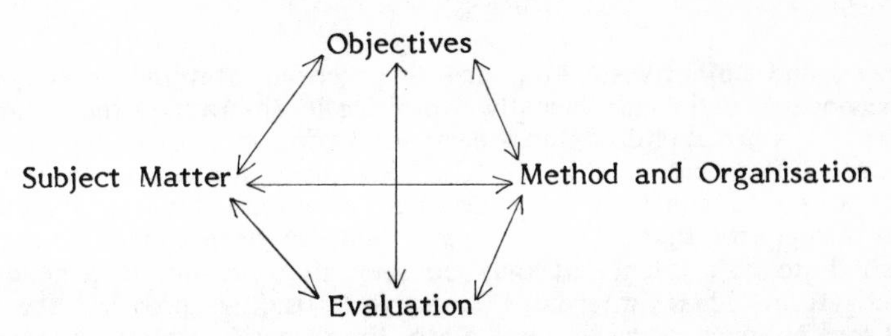

Taba points out that this design describes the interrelationship of these four elements but she stresses that for the curriculum developer it raises four questions:

- what is to be done?
- what subject matter is to be used?
- what methods and organisation are to be employed?
- how are the results of be appraised?

While this model of curriculum is still widely employed, Nicholls and Nicholls (1978:21) argue for 'a much wider and more comprehensive approach to diagnosis, an analysis of all the factors which make up the total situation followed by the use of knowledge and insights derived from this analysis in curriculum planning'. They stress the need for situation analysis to be a major stage in curriculum development and suggest the following model.

Figure 3:2 A Curriculum Model, following Nicholls and Nicholls

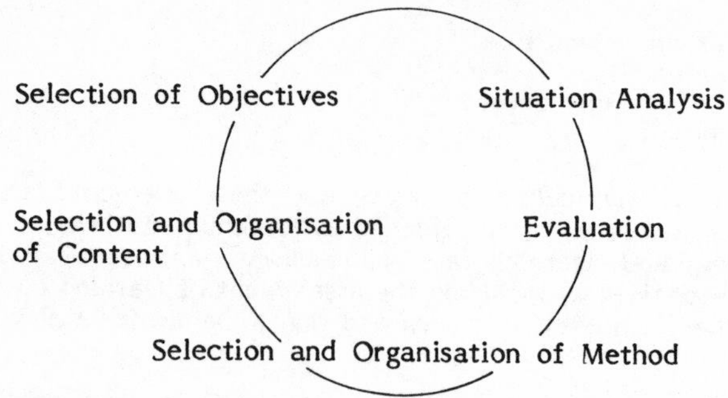

However, this cyclical model implies that everything occurs in sequence, whereas the selection and organisation of content and method may occur concurrently during curriculum design.

Having briefly considered the concept of curriculum and some of the elements that comprise it, these categories are now discussed in more detail.

Aims and Objectives: Aims are very general statements of goals and purposes and they are usually expressed in abstract terms. They often provide a broad philosophical perspective for the curriculum and Davies (1976:12) considers that an aim 'attempts to give both shape and direction to a set of more detailed intentions for the future'. He also suggests that an aim is 'an ideal, an aspiration, a direction in which to go'. Hence it may be seen that an aim is a general and long-term idea, whereas 'objectives' usually provide the actual direction over a more immediate time span. Objectives are more specific statements of the philosophical perspective and may be viewed as the means to achieving the long term intention. Objectives may be expressed along two continua from general to specific, or from long-term to medium-term to short-term. Another curriculum theorist, Wheeler (1967), refers to ultimate, mediate and proximate goals; with the ultimate goals being synonymous with the aims, the mediate ones relating to the specific development of a subject and the proximate relating to the direction of the individual lesson.

The pre-specification of aims and objectives, or whatever terminology is employed, is the result of educators attempting to provide direction for the development of the curriculum at every level. However, the desirability of providing such direction is open to considerable question, especially since it proposes a teacher-centred learning model and this is not necessarily acceptable to educators of adults (see Robinson and Taylor, 1983). Increasingly, learner-centred approaches are gaining acceptance, especially with adult educators, since it is now recognised that education is fundamentally about learning rather than teaching and that, ultimately, the teacher is not essential to the learning process. Hence, there has been a movement towards expressing objectives in learning rather than teaching terms, for example:

- educational objectives (Bloom et al, 1956)
- instructional objectives (Mager, 1975)
- behavioural objectives (Reilly, 1975)
- performance objectives (Davies, 1976)
- expressive objectives (Eisner in Popham, 1969)

It will be appreciated therefore, that a number of different approaches might be recommended for producing specific objectives, since all of these stress learning outcomes. However, there are marked similarities between the first four of the aforementioned types, since all suggest that the objectives should specify the intended behaviour that the student should attain, the standards to be achieved and the conditions under which the behaviour will be manifest. It will be emphasized later in this section that some scholars consider that such precise prescription of desired behaviour is contrary to the ideals of adult education, unless these prescriptions have been negotiated between teacher and learner in advance, so that expressive objectives are much more in keeping with these ideals. Before discussing expressive objectives it is necessary to explore some of the literature on objectives that relate to other four types.

Educational and behavioural objectives may be specified in all three domains, ie cognitive, affective and psychomotor, although they most frequently relate to the cognitive. Bloom et al (1956) devised one of the most well known taxonomies of educational objectives in this domain, whilst Krathwohl et al (1964) discussed one for the affective domain. More recently, Harrow (1972) and Simpson (1966) have been responsible for designing taxonomies in the psychomotor domain and while the cognitive is used most frequently, all three will be discussed here.

Bloom et al suggest that there are six levels of knowledge:

- knowledge of specifics eg terminology, facts
- comprehension eg recipient is able to understand communication on specific topics
- application eg ability to utilise specific knowledge to solve a problem
- analysis eg ability to break down material into component parts and to detect interrelationships
- synthesis eg ability to draw together the parts to form a whole

- evaluation eg ability to judge the value or purpose of ideas.

Bloom and his associates (1956: 15-16) acknowledge that in producing the taxonomy in the cognitive domain they had been unable to produce a classification system that allowed for sharp distinctions in behaviour to be drawn and they recognised that complex behaviour is more than the sum of the more simple elements. That they placed so much emphasis on behaviour, even though they were writing in the cognitive domain, may now seem somewhat surprising, but this emphasis may have resulted in the popularity of the concept of behavioural objectives and the decline in emphasis being given to the term educational objectives. This taxonomy may be useful for the teacher practitioner to judge the appropriate levels of knowledge to which she should help the students aspire. The teacher practitioner utilising the nursing, midwifery or health visiting process will appreciate the need to help students utilise knowledge at all levels if they are to acquire a professional approach to practice.

In this first study Bloom and associates concentrated upon the cognitive domain but, subsequently, Krathwohl, Bloom et al (1964) produced a second taxonomy in the affective domain and since teacher practitioners are involved in helping students acquire attitudes appropriate to working with people in stressful situations this taxonomy is included here:

- receiving eg awareness, willingness to receive
- responding eg ability and willingness to respond and participate with others
- valuing eg acceptance and commitment to values
- organisation eg organising values into a system and recognition of the more important elements
- characterisation eg the unique set of values that make up individuality, a philosophy of life.

It will be noted by teacher practitioners that this relates closely to values for professional practice. Krathwohl and his colleagues relate this taxonomy to the process of internalisation and they (1964:44) claim that 'as internalisation progresses, the learner comes to attend to phenomena, to respond to them, to value and to conceptualise them'. They recognised that this process is akin to socialisation although not synonymous with it.

Bloom and his colleagues did not wish this separate analysis into cognitive and affective domains to be regarded as indicating that they drew a fundamental separation between them, rather they were seeking to provide a theoretical framework for educational objectives. Teacher practitioners should not, therefore, overlook the basic unity of the two domains but it will be recognised immediately that the setting of affective/evaluative objectives in this manner may be interpreted as a form of indoctrination. But since professionalism itself, as discussed earlier, has a moral basis, it might be argued that no profession should admit new recruits who have not had the opportunity to consider ethical issues underlying the practice of the profession and who embrace certain of them which they regard as basic to their own practice. Since nurses, midwives and health visitors are required to interact and care for patients and clients with impartiality it could be maintained that it would be immoral to admit to practice those whose standards and values inhibit this. Thus teacher practitioners should be aware of objectives in the affective domain and be prepared to utilise them appropriately in the teaching and learning transaction, since attitudes and values are included in some of the syllabi of their professions.

However, the teacher practitioner is also a teacher of skills and while Bloom and his associates never devised a taxonomy of educational objectives in the psychomotor domain, at least two have been devised since the publication of this work. Harrow (1972) suggested that there are six levels of skill:

-	reflex movements	eg	to flex
-	basic fundamental movements	eg	to crawl
-	perceptual abilities	eg	to catch
-	physical abilities	eg	to move precisely
-	skilled movements	eg	to type
-	non-discursive communication	eg	utilisation of skilled movements to express emotion

While this taxonomy is a useful starting point in thinking about the psychomotor domain, Simpson's (1966) taxonomy may be more useful to the teacher practitioner.

-	perceptual ability	eg	awareness through the senses
-	readiness	eg	knowing what to do and how to do it
-	learning parts of a skill	eg	by imitation, practice
-	habitualisation	eg	internalisation of a skill
-	performing complex motor acts	eg	automatic performance of co-ordinated skill
-	adapting and originating	eg	devising individual ways to skill performance according to individual perception

It may thus be seen from Simpson's classification that one element in skills teaching is that of breaking the skill into its component parts and helping the learner with each part. Adult learners should be allowed to practise skills at their own pace, as will be discussed in a later chapter. The final point that Simpson makes is that the highest level in skill performance is that of adaptation, so that it would be unwise for the teacher practitioner to expect that students will imitate her and then continue to perform the skill in precisely the way that it has been demonstrated.

Some educationalists, eg Eisner (in Popham 1969:8) consider behavioural objectives compatible with training since they provide 'specific types of behavioural responses to specific stimuli or situations,' but that these are not suitable for education. He (1969:8) considers that the process 'enables individuals to behave intelligently through the exercise of judgments in situations that demand reflection, appraisal and choice among alternative courses of action'. Therefore, it is likely that the educational process will produce different learning outcomes for individual students. In such instances, behavioural objectives may be considered inappropriate and their morality needs to be questioned; expressive objectives, therefore, are more appropriate and might be employed. These are in marked contrast to behavioural ones since they describe an educational encounter in which the student and teacher engage but do not specify its outcome. Eisner (in Popham 1969:16) suggests that expressive objectives provide both teacher and student with the opportunity to explore issues that are significant to them but it is not prescriptive, since the individuality of the persons and the uniqueness of the experience should not result in homogeneity. Expressive objectives are not, therefore, intended as a common measure of learning outcomes but a basis upon which lessons may be planned. They are, therefore, useful in the individualised learning situation where the teacher practitioner and the learner may share their experiences to their mutual enrichment, although it needs to be recognised that the responsibility for the teaching and learning transaction must remain with the teacher practitioner.

While the morality of behavioural objectives has been questioned, there is a sense in which mutually agreed behavioural objectives may have a place in skills training, but even these require negotiation. Hence in the education and training of professional practitioners a combination of behavioural and expressive objectives may be approriate, although the place of the latter should be more significant than that of the former.

Content: In professional education the content of the curriculum should comprise the knowledge, skills and attitudes considered appropriate for practice. In some situations the role for which the learner is being prepared has been fully analysed and the different elements of the content identified and in these instances the curriculum may itself be based upon numerous specific objectives that will form a rationale for content selection. Alternatively, the curriculum developers may have relied solely upon aims, or general objectives, in producing an outline curriculum. In which case, the decision about what content to include, eg. appropriate knowledge, skills and attitudes, and how to structure it, eg. multi-disciplinary or interdisciplinary, thematic or modular, is the responsibility of the local school of nursing, midwifery or college department. When the selection of content has been made it is submitted to the statutory body for approval, which is an element in the validation process which includes inspection of the school of nursing, or midwifery or college, etc. Once that validation exercise has been undertaken the school or college is licensed to mount the course of preparation of new recruits to the profession for a specific time, often five years, so that the actual validated course might be a static entity only during that period. However, professional practice is frequently changing and teacher practitioners are in an ideal situation to ensure that new developments in professional practice are reflected in new submissions for validation, so that it may be seen that the teacher practitioner should be helping to ensure that every new curriculum should be relevant to professional practice. This also indicates that often curriculum content follows professional practice rather than vice versa.

Since students differ in personality, ability, experiences and knowledge their learning needs during their professional preparation differ, so that the actual content of any teaching and learning session is rarely prescribed by either the document that was submitted for validation or the organisers of the course. Hence, the teacher practitioner has responsibility for the selection of content in the individual sessions that she teaches. This is a responsibility that she may exercise in a variety of ways, including discussing with the student the areas that she considers should be covered. However she approaches it, there are some teaching sessions in which she is responsible for structuring the content, so that it is most easily learned by the student and there are a number of points that she may find useful when doing this. The content should:

- be seen to be relevant to the student
- move from the known to the unknown
- develop from the simple to the complex
- develop from the concrete to the abstract
- develop from the particular to the general
- commence with the whole, sub-divide into the parts and then resynthesize into the whole

Thus it may be seen here that the teacher practitioner will be able to relate theory to practice and practice to theory. In addition, it will be noted that this sequencing fits into the experiential learning cycle that is discussed elsewhere in this text. Overall, it is suggested that this approach forms the basis of student-centred teaching that is relevant to the work of the teacher practitioner. If the teacher practitioner concentrates on the process of the teaching and learning transaction then the successful outcome of the process is more likely to be achieved.

Methods: Few curricula specify the precise teaching and learning strategies to be employed by the teaching staff responsible for their implementation, although some statutory bodies, eg. the English National Board, require information about the methods that are to be employed when the submission of the course is made. However, the type of information required is of a general, rather than specific, nature so that the teacher usually has freedom of choice in deciding what approaches to utilise. Naturally, the teacher's own philosophy and experience in teaching adults will influence the methods utilised but the learning objectives, the content and the situation will also exercise considerable constraint upon the methods finally selected. The fifth chapter of this book is devoted to teaching methods so that further discussion on the actual methods will be deferred.

Evaluation: The term 'evaluation' means 'to place a value upon' so that in the educational context it tends to be restricted to curriculum development, while the word 'assessment' usually refers to the process of appraising students' abilities and this latter term is discussed fully in the sixth chapter.

Curriculum evaluation is a complex topic and space forbids detailed explanation of it here. Nevertheless, it may be seen from Figure 3:2 that curriculum evaluation involves an examination of the appropriateness of the aims, objectives and content and of the effectiveness and appropriateness of the methods employed. The complexity of the subject becomes more apparent when it is recognised that there may be no agreed philosophy underlying all aspects of the course, little way of assessing the appropriateness of all the content to the work situation and only subjective means of measuring the effectiveness of the teaching methods employed or the learning experiences provided. Hence, there are no objective and universal standards of measurement and no accepted baselines from which the learning outcome can be appraised. Thus, the attractiveness of behavioural objectives might be seen, since they might be regarded as a baseline from which the effectiveness of the teaching and learning may be measured. But, as will be demonstrated in the following chapter, behaviourism provides a false definition of learning, so that it is ultimately a weak support in the process of evaluation. More recently, the concept of illuminative evaluation has become more popular with curriculum theorists: this approach enables the evaluator to make his own subjective assessment of the process which he has observed and which allows the recipient of the evaluation to make his own decision about the curriculum (see Hamilton 1976:39).

Frequently, tutors seek an evaluation from their students of the course in which they have participated and this is often conducted at the end of the course by means of questionnaire. While there is a certain value in this approach, it must be remembered that this is an immediate assessment of a process which may also have long term effects, so that it may be more relevant to evaluate the course immediately after it has been completed and again a few months later when the new recruits are fully established in practice.

Each of the elements of the curriculum have now been examined briefly in order to highlight the theory underlying the course in which the teacher practitioner is involved. Since she is a teacher, as well as a practitioner, it is also essential that she understands the way in which learning programmes are designed.

II The Design of Learning Experiences

The teacher practitioner is responsible for designing learning experiences but, unfortunately, much of the literature on this topic fails to distinguish between designing institutional provision of education and individual learning experiences wherever these occur. Nevertheless, the programme building models designed by some American scholars have relevance for teachers concerned with either type of provision, so that some aspects of these are now considered.

From a large volume of literature published on the topic in the United States, there are according to Long (1983:158) four most frequently cited stages in designing a learning experience:

- determine the training needs
- design the programme
- provide the instruction
- evaluate the programme.

It may be seen that these four points have considerable similarity with the different aspects of the curriculum discussed above, especially if the teacher's objectives are to endeavour to respond to the students's needs. However, it will be noted that these four points assume that the educational activity is teacher initiated and designed. This is less true of the model constructed by Knowles (1980:223-3), whose learner-centred model is outlined below:

- set a climate for learning
- establish a structure for mutual planning
- diagnose needs for learning
- formulate directions (objectives) for learning
- design a pattern of learning experiences
- manage the execution of the learning experiences
- evaluate the results
- rediagnose the learning needs

This approach relates more closely to the one advocated here than to the teacher initiated one mentioned above. It will be seen immediately the Knowles' first step is very similar to that discussed in the previous chapter, when the importance of establishing a good relationship with the student was highlighted. However, it is the second point that requires emphasis here: while the teacher practitioner may know in her own mind what she thinks the student ought to learn, she must also recognise that as an adult (and maybe as an experienced nurse) the student might also know what she would like, or thinks, she needs to learn. Therefore, it is maintained that the design of the student's learning experience should emerge after a period of mutual planning. This does not mean that the teacher practitioner merely provides what the student wishes to learn, but that in a negotiated situation both participants plan the learning experience. Hence, the diagnosis of learning needs and the formulation of learning objectives may emerge from a mutual planning exercise. This spirit of mutuality should, provided that the interpersonal relationship initially established is maintained, prevail through all the stages of the learning experiences that the teacher practitioner provides for the student.

Long (1983:164) claims that no research known to him has actually tested Knowles' model, but Jarvis and Gibson (1980:71-4) discovered that practical work teachers and student district nurses, who did not undertake a period of mutual planning, often had completely different aims for the same period of professional practical experience. Hence, this time of professional practice had not resulted in such a rich teaching and learning experience as it might have done had there been some joint planning. Knowles does employ two other concepts in his model of designing learning experiences that require further elucidation: needs and diagnosis. Hence, the next two sections of this chapter will consider these concepts.

III The Concept of Need

It will have become apparent from the above discussion that the learner and the teacher practitioner may perceive the student's needs in differing ways. This indicates one of the major problems of the concept of 'need' in education; it is used in a variety of ways by different participants in the educational process and even by different scholars. Many teacher practitioners will be familiar with Maslow's famous hierarchy of needs:

Figure 3.3 Maslow's Hierarchy of Needs

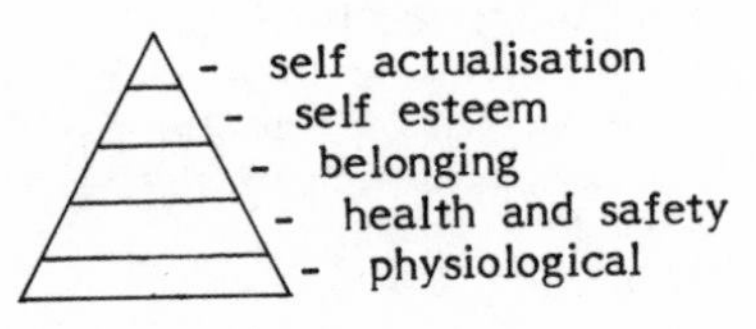

While this model has proved a helpful starting point for many discussions about the subject, it certainly does not exhaust the debate (see Jarvis 1983b:14-19). Additionally, Hirst and Peters (1970:33) suggest that there are needs of a diagnostic, biological, psychological basic and functional type, whilst Bradshaw (1972) considers that there are normative, felt, expressed and comparative needs. Hence, it may be seen that the concept itself is complex and confused.

Lawson (1975:37) tried to clarify the debate when he suggested that 'a deficiency (that) can be remedied by the help of some educational process' may be regarded as an educational need. This is a useful definition in many ways because it specifies a type of need but 'education' is a much more difficult term to define. Even more problematic in this definition is the implication that educational processes are always designed to remedy a deficiency rather than to respond to wants or interests. More recently, it has been suggested by some writers, eg. Illich (1977), Armstrong (1982), that the concept is ideological. The reason for this accusation is that learning needs are frequently defined from above, ie. it is the teacher or professional body which defines the need, rather than from below, ie. the learner. This accusation certainly appears to have some validity since it is usually assumed that the professional is the person to diagnose and the client/patient is a passive recipient of the diagnosis.

This also appears to be true for traditional education, and it might be argued that in the case of children that there is every justification for this approach. A similar argument might be presented in professional education, since the qualified professional should know what the new recruit needs. However, many of the students that teacher practitioners teach are already experienced professional practitioners, eg. the community teaching midwife may be teaching someone who is a registered general nurse and the fieldwork teacher's student may be both a registered general nurse and midwife. Hence, it is necessary for the teacher practitioner to recognise that the student may be very aware of deficiences that she may have, ie. felt needs, and that she may be prepared to express them provided that the relationship established between herself and the teacher practitioner is conducive to mutual planning. In these instances, needs are not ideological in the manner that Illich and Armstrong suggest, since they are not concerned with control. But at the same time the teacher practitioner should be in a position to perceive needs of which the student may be unaware.

IV The Notion of Diagnosis

Knowles refers to this as diagnosing learning needs, whereas other writers, such as Rowntree (1977), discuss a similar concept under the title of formative assessment. Rowntree (1977:121-122) states that formative assessment occurs when the teacher intends to use 'the knowledge he gains about the student .... diagnostically (in helping) the student grow'. Hence, diagnostic appraisal is a teaching tool. It has been suggested elsewhere, (Jarvis, 1979), that if the teacher practitioner is to use the limited time available to her to the best possible advantage, she should undertake a diagnostic appraisal of the student's work very early in the period of time allocated to professional practice.

This approach to diagnosis of needs requires the teacher practitioner and the student to identify jointly those areas in which the student is already proficient and those in which further assistance will be required. Obviously there may be instances where the teacher practitioner wishes to assess the student's level of knowledge, skills and attitudes in order to decide whether she thinks that the student is proficient, since she may have different standards to those of the student. The teacher practitioner would then be in a position to discuss with the learner what she considers to be the student's learning needs and they can then negotiate the areas in which further teaching and learning should occur. Thus it may be seen that since the adult learner brings certain skills and experiences to the individualised teaching and learning situation the programme should be prepared to respond to the teaching and learning needs jointly agreed upon by both teacher practitioner and student. Diagnosis should be undertaken during the early stage of the teaching and learning programme and it should then become an on-going process. Whilst the teacher practitioner should regard herself as a diagnostician she should not automatically or autocratically prescribe the educational remedy for the diagnosis. She should, however, be prepared to discuss her diagnosis with the learner, who might also have felt needs in these areas or even disagree with the teacher practitioner's diagnosis and wish to discuss it further. Therefore, the teaching and learning programme may be something that is both mutually agreed but flexible enough to allow for development or modification, depending upon the learning needs of the student as perceived by both the learner and the teacher practitioner. The idea of mutual planning is also known as a negotiated curriculum, but the difference between it and many other negotiated curricula is that in this instance the negotiation should be an on-going process throughout the whole of the teaching and learning period and not something that occurs once only at the outset of the programme.

Whilst 'needs' are a useful basis for programme planning the teacher practitioner and the student must ensure that all aspects of the content of the curriculum are covered during the professional practical experience and that they are dealt with in the appropriate depth and breadth in relation to those needs.

V Implementing and Managing a Learning Programme

From what has been written thus far in this chapter it may be seen that in individualised teaching and learning in the education of adults it is advocated that the planning process should be a mutual undertaking between the teacher practitioner and the learner. However, it is recognised that the approach suggested here is an ideal one and that it is not always possible to implement. On occasions, the teacher practitioner may have had little time to discuss everything with the learner. On other occasions, she may endeavour to act independently of the learner for a variety of reasons, although it is emphasized here that this should be the exception rather than the rule. However, even in this situation of mutuality, it must be recognised that it is still the teacher practitioner's responsibilty to provide the teaching or facilitation through which the learning may occur. Davies (1971:22-30) equates the teacher to a manager and he coined the phrase teacher manager and while this phrase is not totally acceptable here, since it implies a form of authority other than that of the professional, it is realistic to recognise that there are sufficient similarities between the ideas of teacher and manager to allow for comparison. Davies, for instance, points out that there are four management functions that are appropriate to teaching: planning, organising, leading and controlling. Thus far it has been advocated that the planning should be a mutual exercise, when ever possible, between two human beings each seeking to maximise the potential of the interaction. Clearly, when the teacher practitioner has resources at her disposal she should organise them in order of achieve the objectives that have been agreed. The methods that she chooses to teach and the teaching aids that she prepares may all be regarded as part of the process. Davies suggests that teaching may be related to motivating, encouraging and inspiring learners, and in this sense, it relates both to the quality of the interpersonal relationship established and to the professionalism of the teacher practitioner which may inspire the learner to seek to achieve similar standards. Finally, Davies equates controlling to monitoring the learning and adjusting the process if it is not as efficient as it might be. In this manner, the teacher practitioner may be regarded as managing the learning experience but perhaps Knowles' (1980:239) description of the teacher is a little more appropriate to the role of the teacher practitioner in implementing and managing the learning experience.

> The role of the teacher in this phase .... is to serve both as a strong procedural technician .... suggesting the most effective ways the students can help in executing the decisions (how to implement strategies of learning into effective learning situations) - and as a resource person or coach, who provides substantial information regarding the subject matter of the unit, possible techniques and available materials where needed. The leader can also perform a useful 'threading' function, providing the connective tissue or transitional commentary from one unit to the next.

While Knowles acknowledges that the teacher does manage the teaching and learning transaction he emphasizes the role of the learner far more than does Davies and is, therefore, much more in accord with the approach to teaching and learning that is advocated here. Even so, it cannot be emphasized enough that however successful the interpersonal relation between the teacher practitioner and learner, the former remains responsible for achieving effectively the overall aim of this element in the professional preparation of each student.

Conclusion

This chapter has begun to explore some of the main issues that indicate the design of a learning programme and perhaps can be summarised by expanding Knowles' "andragogical model" of the teacher whose role is to:

- set the climate, by establishing good interpersonal relations from the outset
- establish a structure of mutual planning, so that
    a. the overall aim of the professional practice is recognised
    b. procedures for discussion about progress are decided
    c. procedures for planning the professional experience are agreed upon
- diagnose learning needs by
    a. listening to the learner express the needs that she recognises
    b. assessing her practice and diagnosing her strengths and weaknesses
    c. agreeing together on the areas of strength and need
- formulate objectives for learning, by mutual planning
- design a pattern of learning experiences, by
    a. selecting appropriate teaching methods/learning experiences
    b. effective utilisation of all resources, including colleagues and their caseloads, as appropriate
- manage the learning experiences, by
    a. implementing the plan
    b. monitoring the process

- evaluate the results, by

  a. discussion with the learner about both the process and her own assessment of what she has gained
  b. observation of the product, where appropriate

- rediagnose the learning needs, by

  a. listening to the learner express the needs that she recognises
  b. assessing her practice and diagnosing the strength and needs
  c. agreeing together on the areas of strength and need

Thereafter the process should begin again, so that the teacher practitioner is continually redesigning the plans for the programme to ensure that by the end of the period of professional practice its overall aim will have been achieved.

Chapter Four

ADULT LEARNING

Learning may be defined as 'the acquisition of knowledge, skills and attitudes by study, experience or teaching' (Jarvis 1983a:5). It may be noted immediately that this definition differs from many others which emphasise a change in behaviour e.g. learning is 'a relatively permanent change in behaviour that occurs as a result of practice' (Hilgard and Atkinson 1967:270). This latter definition highlights only behaviour modification whereas the former is less restrictive, embracing the cognitive, affective and psychomotor domains. Learning is, therefore, a broader phenomenon than that implied by some conventional definitions.

That adults have ability to learn has never been denied although it has been assumed frequently that learning is mainly undertaken in childhood and that the ability to learn, and also intelligence, decline as the adult ages. Research in recent years has, however, suggested that the age limit on learning performance may not occur before 75 years (Cross 1981:154), so that the adage that 'old dogs cannot learn new tricks' is a myth that needs to be laid to rest. However, it has also been shown that the methods by which adults learn change, so that it is incumbent for the teacher practitioner to be aware of recent research findings in this area in order to ensure that she becomes a more effective teacher.

Learning, then, is a lifelong process, but it is useful to know some of the theoretical perspectives about it, so that the first part of this chapter contains a very brief summary of some of the main theories. The weaknesses of some of these approaches are highlighted in an examination of an experiential learning cycle. Thereafter, the concepts of adulthood and adult development are discussed and it is recognised that adults bring different characteristics to bear upon learning.

Learning in the cognitive, affective and psychomotor domains is considered thereafter, and the chapter concludes with a summary of those elements discussed herein which are known to enhance or inhibit adult learning.

I. Theories of Learning

A number of theories of learning have been propounded over the years. All of them have value but one of the major weaknesses that many of them have is that the research upon which they are based has been conducted with animals rather than developed with adults, consequently they are not completely satisfactory as explanations of adult learning. Three broad areas are mentioned here: connectionism, conditioning and gestalt theory.

Connectionism: This is frequently referred to as 'stimulus-response' learning and was developed by Thorndike (1928), whose research was conducted with cats, dogs and chickens. His research led him to those three laws of learning, which he believed applied equally well to humans as to animals. These are the laws of:

- effect; the bond between stimulus and response is strengthened or weakened because of the level of emotive satisfaction that accompanies the action
- exercise; repetition of meaningful actions results in substantial learning
- readiness; if the organism is ready for the connection then the result is pleasurable and learning is increased but, if not, then the opposite result occurs.

There are elements of learning in these laws that it is important for teacher practitioners to consider, e.g.,

- the greater the pleasure obtained from the learning experience, the more learning that will occur
- the more meaningful the act to the student, the greater will be the resultant learning
- practice makes perfect, provided that the action is seen to be meaningful.

Pleasure and relevance are important elements in learning and in the teaching and learning transaction both should occur if learning is to be enhanced.

Conditioning: Both forms of conditioning are well known - classical and operant. Classical conditioning is associated with the work of Pavlov, who demonstrated that behaviour could be initiated by a stimulus. He showed that a dog could be made to salivate to the sound of a bell provided that on a number of previous occasions the sound had been presented simultaneously with food. However, salivation will only occur for as long as the dog associates the sound with the food. Hence, it may be seen that in classical conditioning the process commences with an already well established response to a stimulus and the response is then associated with a different stimulus. This process occurs in therapy, when the patient may be conditioned by the therapist to acquire approved behavioural responses to specific stimuli, but it does appear to be a matter of reflex rather than cognitive learning. Perhaps Skinner's operant conditioning, equally well known, has more applicability to education. He experimented with both rats and pigeons and demonstrated that by rewarding acceptable behaviour both could be taught to perform the type of behaviour that the experimenter wished them to learn; even relatively complicated behaviour could be taught by rewarding correct performance at each stage in its development. From his experiments, Skinner concluded that:

- learning could be maximised by positive reinforcement

- each stage in a complicated process needs to be restricted and grow out of previously learned behaviour

- reward should immediately be given after correctly learned behaviour

- the learner should be provided with the opportunity to discover behaviour that is not rewarded.

In this above formulation, it is possible to see how skills might be taught by breaking the procedure into a number of manageable sections, and helping the student learn each stage in the sequence by individually rewarding each correct performance. Reward should be forthcoming in the shape of praise etc., which is a substitute for the sweets sometimes given to children for good behaviour. In the same way as skills can be taught by this approach, so cognitive and affective response can be learned. However, the extent to which conditioning is an educational process is open to debate. Nevertheless, it is a method of maximising learning and positive re-inforcement is a weapon in every teacher's armoury, and it is a very important element in individualised teaching and learning in order to enhance the personal relationship that has been established between the teacher practitioner and the learner. Additionally, it may be seen that operant conditioning may occur both in programmed learning and therapy.

Gestalt Psychology: Gestalt psychologists have tended to use apes or gorillas in their research and they have shown that these animals have been able to grasp patterns of actions when seeking to solve a problem. From these experiments it has been possible to suggest that the solutions:

- appear to occur by inspiration or insight
- occur as a result of perceived relationships within a given situation
- are permanent to that situation.

Clearly some people do appear to respond to learning situations best when they have a holistic perspective, so that this approach to learning might well reflect one learning style. Hence, it may be seen that it may be beneficial for adult students to be presented with a meaningful whole in the first instance rather than isolated elements.

It would be possible to extend this discussion considerably but this is not within the scope of this small text, although further references are given in the recommended reading list at the end of this book.

II The Learning Cycle

From the above section, it may be concluded that the more developed the species of animal, the greater the theory of learning appears to rely upon the active involvement of the learner. Hence, it is suggested here that human learning frequently involves something other than a reflex action acquired in response to a stimulus, but that it demands a process of active thought by the learner. This active involvement may occur in the form of reflection upon an experience, a problem or a situation and this may be presented in the form of a learning cycle. Much of the work on learning cycles has been developed by exponents of experiential learning, although it is maintained here that the learning process is similar irrespective of the dimension in which the experience occurs. Additionally, it is important to recognise that there is an inter-relationship between the cognitive, affective and psychomotor dimensions and that changes in one of them may, but need not necessarily, result in changes in the other two.

One learning cycle frequently cited is that devised by Kolb and Fry (1975:33-7) and it is presented here in this simple, initial formulation.

Figure 4.1. An Experiential Learning Cycle - following Kolb and Fry

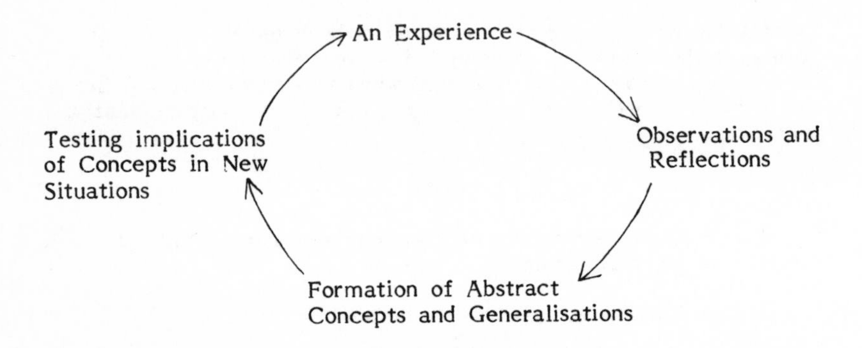

Any experience occurs within a complex integration of all three dimensions, i.e., cognitive, affective and psychomotor, with possibly one of them being dominant. The experience may be facilitated by the teacher practitioner although it may occur in the events of everyday living or working. Students may observe a situation, reflect upon it and learn and the teacher practitioner may remain oblivious that a learning situation has occurred.

Hence, it may be seen that the human being does not merely receive a stimulus and respond to it - he has to think about it! Reflection is a significant element in human learning and one that it is important for the teacher practitioner to take into consideration in providing students with the opportunities to learn about aspects of the practical situation. However, reflection itself is not a simple process that occurs automatically or only at one level. Mezirow (1981:24) has suggested that there are seven levels of reflectivity:

- reflectivity; awareness of seeing, thinking or acting
- affective reflectivity; awareness of feelings
- discriminant reflectivity; assessment of the efficiency of reflection in the context of reality
- judgmental reflectivity; being aware of the subjective value judgments about reflections

- conceptual reflectivity; assessment of whether the theoretical concepts employed are sufficient to explain perceived reality

- psychic reflectivity; considering the adequacy of the evidence employed to explain perceived reality

- theoretical reflectivity; awareness that taken-for-granted assumptions may be less than sufficient to explain perceived reality.

Mezirow suggests that the first four of these levels of reflectivity are of a lower order than the remaining three, so that the former ones are regarded by him as 'consciousness' while the latter are regarded as 'critical-conciousness'. Becoming critically aware is an important stage in the development of any person, especially those being educated to enter nursing, midwifery and health visiting. As one of the main aims of education, teacher practitioners should strive to produce critically aware fellow practitioners rather than recruits to the profession who merely conform to the theory and practice with which they are presented.

It may be seen that reflection not only occurs at the second stage in the learning cycle but it also occurs in the third stage of formulating abstract concepts, so that it must be recognised that the learning cycle in Figure 4.1 is an over-simplification of reality. Nevertheless, opportunity should be given by teacher practitioners for students to reflect upon their experiences and try to draw theoretical conclusions about them, conclusions about which the learner may still wish to be critical. Finally, the learner has to test the implications of the learning in new situations. Such a test may itself become a new experience that reactivates the whole process once again or it may become new knowledge that the learner then commits to memory, etc.

In precisely the same way the experiences may pose a problem for the student who may then endeavour to solve it through a process of reflection that leads to possible solutions which need testing, etc. Hence, both active learning and problem solving may be viewed as similar processes which actually continue throughout the life-span. The process of reflection is, therefore, quite critical to learning and it is one that must influence the way that the teacher practitioner performs her role. For instance, she must:

- be prepared to let the learner think things out for herself

- ask sufficient, relevant questions to encourage the process of reflection

- allow the learner to think things through at her own pace

- not seem too anxious that the learner should actually reach a conclusion

- not expect that the learner will necessarily arrive at the same conclusion as she herself has reached

- not pressurize the student to reject solutions with which she disagrees.

By this approach the teacher practitioner demonstrates recognition of the adulthood and maturity of the learner and encourages autonomy and independence which are both essential attributes in the practice of nursing, midwifery and health visiting.

III Adult Learning

The concept of adulthood has excercised the minds of a number of writers on adult education, including Knowles (1980) and Paterson (1979). The intricacies of that discussion are not really the concern of this book, but it is very important to recognise in the process of ageing the individual changes physiologically, psychologically and socially. Physiologically the body changes quite dramatically during this process, so that strength, reaction time, learning, vision, respiratory and circulatory functions all eventually undergo decline. Psychologically, the adult continues to develop although no single classification of developmental stages is agreed upon by the scholars. Erikson's (1965) famous eight ages of man indicate four that are significant for all teachers of adults. If this is combined with Schaie's and Parr's thesis (1981) that there are three stages in intellectual development in adulthood, achievement, responsibility and re-integration, and only one in adolescence, acquisition, the following table may be constructed:

Table 4.1. Adult Development and Learning

Age	Characteristics	Cognitive Development
Adolescence	Ego identity versus role diffusion	Acquisition
Early adulthood	Intimacy versus isolation	Achievement
Middle adulthood	Generativity versus stagnation	Responsibilty
Late adulthood	Integrity versus despair	Re-integration

Thus it may be seen that in different stages in the life cycle the individual has different orientations to learning and different perceptions of the self. Each of the experiences of life expand the individual's reservoir of knowledge and understanding, so that it is now claimed that crystallised intelligence, influenced by education and experience, expands between the ages of 19 and 61 years, whereas fluid intelligence, biologically determined intellectual ability, declines during the same period (Cross 1981:162). These two changes may balance each other out, so that adults can continue to learn effectively throughout their working life, although the method of learning might well change significantly. Hence, it may be necessary to take these changes into consideration when developing an understanding and a theoretical perspective on adult learning. This is precisely what Knowles (1980) has attempted to do in developing his well known theory of andragogy - the art and science of helping adults learn. Knowles highlights four significant assumptions in andragogy:

- the learner; moves from dependence to independence during maturation
- the learner's experience; becomes an increasingly rich resource for learning
- readiness to learn; adults are ready to learn material relevant to their life situation
- orientation to learning; adults wish to apply what they learn, so that education should be organised around comprehensive categories.
(Knowles 1980:43-44)

Knowles' claims about andragogy have been widely debated in both North America and the United Kingdom (see Jarvis 1983b for a summary). While many of the criticisms levelled at this theory undoubtedly contain substance (e.g. does the learner necessarily become more independent during maturation? is this an actual theory of learning at all?), the very persistence of the theory indicates that it embodies some truths that reflect the experiences of educators of adults. Hence, andragogy may indicate an ideology about teaching and learning with adults that may lead adult educators to produce an environment that enhances adults' learning processes. Most certainly these four significant assumptions are relevant to the work of the teacher practitioner in the majority of situations.

IV Cognitive Learning Styles

Earlier in this chapter it was suggested that some learners may be more effective if they start with a holistic perspective and in the previous section it was indicated that as individuals age so their approaches to learning change. Hence, it may be recognised that different people have different styles of learning, something that it is important for teacher practitioners to ascertain with their own students. It is well known, for instance, that some people learn more effectively by reading, whilst others prefer to see or hear in order to maximise their acquisition of knowledge, etc. There have been a number of different formulations of learning styles (see Knox 1977:447-449, Jarvis 1983b:83-87) and since the teacher practitioner should be aware of these, some of the major ones are discussed briefly below:

- Concrete versus Abstract; some learners like to start with the concrete situation such as experience, while others prefer to commence with an abstract, theoretical idea

- Converger versus Diverger; the converger is best at abstract conceptualization and active experimentation and in situations where there is a single correct solution, whereas divergers are best at concrete experiences and reflective observation where they can generate ideas and have broad perspectives

- Focusing versus Scanning; focusers examine problems as a totality and generate hypotheses as a result of reflection that may be modified in the light of new information, whereas scanners select one aspect of the problem and assume it is the solution until subsequent information disproves it when they have to recommence the task

- Holistic versus Serialistic; some learners see a phenomenon as a whole while others prefer to string together the parts

- Impulsivity versus Reflectivity; some learners respond first and reflect later while others reflect first and respond later.

Obviously no learner adopts only one or other of these types nor does she function entirely at the extreme of any one of them, but it is useful to be aware of the student's most effective learning style, so that the teacher practitioner may prepare handouts for the student who learns best by reading, cassette tapes (especially for community nurses who have to drive between visits) or discussions, for those who are more effective learners from audio input, etc. Additionally, the teacher practitioner may wish to present the whole situation to a holistic learner but not to a serialistic one, etc. Even though there has been a considerable amount of research on learning styles it is also important to recognise that 'there are only hints of association between cognitive style and learning effectiveness for adults' (Knox 1977:448). However, this may be, in part, because less research has actually been conducted with adults than with children in the learning situation. Another important reason for teacher practitioners knowing the preferred learning style of their students is because it may be necessary for them to help their students become more effective in some other styles which would be beneficial to their work situation.

V Learning in the Affective Domain

The affective domain relates to the area of feelings and emotions and it is an aspect of teaching and learning that has received far less emphasis than the cognitive domain. However, it has been recognised in the education of adults that feelings may either enhance or inhibit adult learning, so that it is important to consider this particular aspect here. In addition, it is significant for the teacher practitioner to be aware of education in the affective domain because nursing, midwifery and health visiting are concerned with the care of people and it is necessary for practitioners to have attitudes that enhance the care that they provide. However, it is recognised that this is a very difficult area to explore and ideas like 'acceptable attitudes' are contentious. But their importance in the work of the teacher practitioner is such that they need consideration. This section explores first, the relationships between emotions and learning and, then, the recognition and teaching of attitudes.

Emotions and Learning: A considerable body of knowledge exists in the field of the education of adults about the relationship between feelings and learning and reference to some of it has already been made in this chapter. Considerable emphasis has been placed upon the self-concept of the learner throughout this discussion since it is recognised that there are a number of factors in education that can and do prove stressful to the adult, such as fear that:

- the teaching and learning process will repeat some of the more unhappy experiences that the learners have had at school; this is true both for those who were successful in school and those who were less successful

- the learner role which is not usually associated with adulthood, will conflict with the self-perception

- the learner will not understand or succeed because it is generally, but wrongly, thought that adults are not capable of learning new ideas.

Each of these points relates to the way in which adults are inhibited from learning and progressing because of a lack of belief in themselves. Belbin and Belbin (1972:159) write:

> Adults must believe in themselves as learners and each should be encouraged to relate this concept to the image of himself.
>
> The greatest barrier to training arises from people believing that learning is not for them .... After discovering that they **have** learned, adults begin to see themselves as learners.

In the individualised teaching and learning situation the teacher practitioner is in a position to understand the student's perception of herself and to structure her learning experiences in such a way as to ensure that she regards herself as a successful learner. The teacher practitioner can, therefore:

- help the learner respect herself

- help the learner realise that she is able to reflect upon her experiences and learn from them

- provide feedback to the learner so that she is able to become aware of what she has learned

- enhance the learner's self-image.

Hence, the teacher practitioner is in a position to help the learner to feel more confident about learning which will almost certainly result in more consistent and effective learning.

Learning and Attitudes: An attitude may be defined as 'an enduring system of positive or negative evaluations, emotional feelings and pro or con action tendencies with respect to a social object' (Krech, Crutchfield and Ballachey, 1962:177), so that it may be seen that there is some similarity between attitudes and values. Attitudes have both a cognitive and an affective element and a behavioural tendency, so that while a teacher practitioner is able to observe the student's behaviour in nursing, midwifery or health visiting practice and in interaction with both colleagues and patients she can never be sure that the behaviour always reflects precisely what the student thinks, or feels. At the same time consistent behavioural patterns may be more closely an expression of thoughts and feelings, so that these consistent patterns may actually illustrate the values that a student holds. It will be recalled that Krathwohl (1964) devised a classification scheme for educational objectives in the affective domain: receiving, responding, valuing, organizing and characterizing a value or a value complex. Davies (1976:156) suggests that this is not really a taxonomy of educational objectives but rather a continuum through which individuals pass from awareness to acceptance to preference of a particular value. Knowledge of such a continuum is important for the teacher practitioner who may be required to make a student aware of other values than the ones that she currently displays, e.g., other ways of treating the elderly, the unkempt, other approaches to learning new knowledge, etc. However, it would be indoctrination rather than education if the teacher practitioner deliberately set out with the intention of making the learner hold the same values as she herself had adopted. Nevertheless, there is a place for teaching values and, at least, giving a student the opportunity to consider alternatives. Lewin and his associates (1952) investigated methods of doing this, comparing two different techniques: lecture followed by handout with group discussion. They discovered that group discussion was much more effective than the lecture in producing attitude change and, in a further study, they discovered that a group decision at the end of a group discussion was more effective than individual instruction in producing changes. Hence, it appears that discussion is more effective than instruction in producing attitude change but the group is more effective than the individual. Therefore, the teacher practitioner is at a disadvantage in not having a group of students if she considers that a specific student should reconsider her attitude to any aspect of her work but she can discuss it with the student and then leave it to her to reach her own conclusions.

VI Learning Skills

Teaching psychomotor skills may form a significant element in the work of the teacher practitioner so that it is important to recognise that the same psychological and physiological aspects apply to this domain as they do to the cognitive. Indeed, it is important for the learner to recognise that age is no bar to learning to perform a psychomotor skill at speed: Belbin and Belbin (1972) document the fact that older people can learn skills even if the process might be a little more difficult than it is with teenagers. However, the significant point is that new techniques can be learned by older people, especially if they have ample opportunity to practise them at their own pace in private, and perhaps upon a dummy. However, it must also be recognised that there are problems for adults when they are learning skills. For instance, Smith (1977:198) writes:

> Various authors have found that older trainees have less confidence, take longer to learn and find it difficult to eliminate the mistakes that they are making ..... in addition, the older trainee may be unduly quality conscious, which inhibits the building of skills that depend on speed of action.

Despite this depressing picture Smith suggests that this actually reflects the method of training rather than the acquisition of new skills. He points out that the discovery method, whereby the trainee actually discovers the relevant principles and relationships for himself, is one that enables the older person to acquire relevant skills. However, there are a number of obvious problems about the discovery method in nursing, midwifery and health visiting that need further discussion and this will occur in the following chapter.

In the previous chapter the educational objectives in skills training were discussed and two sets of objectives produced. Harrow's (1972) developmental taxonomy related to maturation but Simpson's (1966) approach outlines various aspects of learning and then proceeds through the stages of the acquisition of a complicated skill leading to its performance in an automatic manner. Clearly automatic behaviour occurs only after practice and this will itself occur only when the learner has the confidence and the supportive environment in which to undertake it. Hence, the teacher practitioner's role may again lie in the creation of a supportive environment in which the student has the confidence to practise. The teacher practitioner's role is, therefore, a very skilled one embracing knowledge, skill and sensitivity through which the learner feels free to practise and to experiment. However, one of the topics of the following chapter is teaching techniques, but before these are discussed it may prove useful to summarise the principles of adult learning discussed in this chapter.

Conclusion

This chapter has provided a broad overview of some of the important elements of adult learning and they are summarised in the following manner.

The adult is:

- able to learn throughout the greater part of his lifespan, so that attention has to be paid to the method of learning as well as the content of what is learned
- continuing to develop and mature so that the reasons why adults learn are significant to the process
- always acquiring experiences which are a rich resource for further learning
- able to learn more effectively when the relevance of what is being learned is recognised
- less able to learn effectively when placed in a stress-creating situation.

In the teaching and learning transaction, the adult:

- should always be treated with dignity and humanity
- should learn in a pleasurable environment
- will learn more effectively if correct learning is rewarded by positive re-inforcement
- will learn more effectively if he has self-confidence
- will learn more effectively if he is free to work at his own pace.

Traditionally theories of learning underplay:

- the humanity of the learner
- the experience of the adult learner

- the place of reflection in the learning process.

Reflection in the adult learning process:

- should be facilitated
- may involve either a conscious or a critically conscious appraisal of the experience
- may develop independence of mind and action.

Skills may be learned by adults through:

- discovery methods
- learning individual stages in a sequence

Hence it may be seen that adults are able to learn throughout most of their lives and that the manner by which the learning process is facilitated may enhance or inhibit the learning. Hence the role of the teacher of adults is quite crucial to this process and the following chapter, therefore, examines methods of teaching adults in an individualised teaching and learning situation.

Chapter Five

TEACHING ADULTS IN INDIVIDUALISED TEACHING AND LEARNING

Teaching is perhaps one of the most widely practised activities in the world: parents teach their children; children teach their parents; adults teach adults in everyday social interaction; teachers teach pupils, etc. In everyday conversation individuals disseminate information and other people learn from it: the latter are, therefore, taught by the former. Hence, it could legitimately be claimed that during an individual's lifetime he will perform the function of teacher on many occasions. However, he will not necessarily be accorded the status of teacher unless he holds a designated role as one, the reason being that the status of teacher is usually restricted to those persons who perform the occupational role of teacher and gain financial reward for teaching students or pupils.

But teaching obviously occurs in contexts other than that of the formal school or college, so that it might be possible to classify teaching in some way according to the type of situation in which it occurs. For instance, parents teach children in an informal context, so that the educational process may be regarded as informal and the teaching viewed as being within the informal mode. By contrast, teachers teach their pupils within the formal structure of the school or college, so that formal education and the teaching may be seen to fall within a formal mode. However, neither of these two types are actually applicable to the situation in which the teacher practitioner teaches her students. Clearly there is a third approach. Recently the concept of non-formal education has been introduced into the world of education and Coombes and Ahmed (1974) define this as:

> any organised, systematic, educational activity carried on outside the framework of the formal system to provide selected types of learning to particular sub-groups in the population, adults as well as children.
>
> (cited in La Belle 1982:161-162)

This type of education obviously falls between the two previous categories mentioned but the above definition does not correlate exactly with the work of the teacher practitioner since she performs her role outside of the formal classroom but within the formal system of professional education. Hence, it is possible to adapt this definition slightly and to suggest that non-formal teaching is 'any organised, systematic, educational activity conducted outside the formal context of the classroom to provide selected types of learning to particular sub-groups in the population, adults as well as children'. Thus it may be claimed that within this definitional framework the teacher practitioner's role may be regarded as a non-formal teaching one. Such an approach has been developed by Srinivasan (1977) within the context of adult learning.

The above definition does not specify what is taught by the teacher practitioner in the context of non-formal education and this is significant because there is often a division made between teaching theory in the formal classroom situation and teaching skills in the non-formal context of professional practice. Hence, the teacher practitioner is sometimes regarded as 'only a teacher of skills'. Such a derogatory categorisation, as implied by this remark, fails to do justice to her role nor does it show awareness of the interrelationship between theory and practice. Nor does such a stance take cognisance of the students' needs. For example, Ogier's (1974) study (cited in Davis 1983) shows that learner nurses expected ward sisters to teach them the theory relating to the skills that they were being taught. The sisters who were rated most highly by the learners related theory to practice on an individualised teaching and learning basis. Hence, this chapter commences with a discussion about this relationship and, thereafter, it explores various styles, methods and aids in teaching.

I Relationship between Theory and Practice

In an earlier chapter it was stated that those teachers who teach theoretical knowledge are ascribed a higher status than those of whom it is claimed teach only skills. It is maintained here, however, that this discussion is over-simplistic and that this status differential is one that reflects a misleading philosophical ideal. Indeed, the teacher practitioner is both a teacher of theory and practice because of the nature of their interrelationships.

The Greeks had the idea that the educated man was one whose life was based upon continual contemplation, for by so doing argued Aristotle the product is a rational individual who both performs good actions and is happy. Hence, for Aristotle, man's actions were performed as a result of rational consideration prior to the act. Ever since that time thinkers have been 'predisposed to find that it was in the capacity for rigorous theory that lay the superiority of man over animals, of civilised men over barbarious, and even of the divine mind over human minds.' (Ryle, 1949:27). Hence, 'to know that' has traditionally been distinguised from 'to know how' and theoretical knowledge been accorded higher status than practical knowledge. Indeed, Ryle (1949: 28) claims:

> Theorists have been so preoccupied with the task of investigating the nature, the source, and the credentials of the theories that we adopt that they have for the most part ignored the question what it is for someone to know how to perform tasks. In ordinary life, on the contrary, as well as in the special business of teaching, we are much more concerned with people's competences than with their cognitive repertoires, with the operations than with the truths that they learn.

Ryle's claims in the above passage are perfectly understandable and reflect a realistic analysis of the current situation, and thinking about 'knowledge how' a task should be performed is a much neglected activity. However, his analysis of this activity led him to make the following claim, that:

> When I do something intelligently, ie thinking what I am doing, I am doing one thing and not two. My performance has a special procedure or manner, not special antecedents.
> (Ryle 1949:32)

Such a conclusion may be considered extreme and may not be universally acceptable, but one of the major merits of this position is that it focuses attention upon the knowledge necessary to undertake the performance of a skill. In the course of his discussion he suggests, for instance, that a person does not have to know the nature of logic before arguing logically, so that 'knowledge that' does not have to precede 'knowledge how', to do so. This is a position that was indicated in the previous chapter when it was suggested that adults may learn psychomotor skills best by first being given the opportunity to explore the relevant principles and relationships for themselves so that they begin to theorise from practice. Thereafter, they can acquire both the 'knowledge how' and, more significantly, the 'knowledge that' it happens. Perhaps, this argument could be extended even further, in accordance with the learning cycle discussed earlier, in order to suggest that 'knowledge why' may logically follow from this. Hence, it may be claimed that in the learning process, 'knowledge how' may most effectively occur first and, indeed, it might be claimed that in many areas of human behaviour it actually occurs automatically first in any case. But it is maintained here that the processes and types of knowledge are different so that this position in no way substantiates Ryle's argument. Why, then, does it appear that 'knowing how' and 'knowing that' are fused into a single process in intelligent action? Perhaps this occurs because the different forms of knowledge may not occur with the same intensity in intelligent behaviour because much of the process appears to be taken for granted in habitualised actions. Berger and Luckmann (1967:71) refer to this process as habitualisation:

> Habitualised actions, of course, retain their meaningful character for the individual although the meanings involved

> become embedded as routines in his general stock of knowledge, taken for granted by him and at hand for his future projects. Habitualisation carries with it an important psychological gain that choices are narrowed. While in theory there are a hundred ways to go about a project of building a canoe out of matchsticks, habitualisation narrows the choice to one. This frees the individual from 'all those decisions,' providing a psychological relief that has its basis in man's undirected instinctual structure.

Berger and Luckmann are pointing to the significant interrelationship of 'knowledge how' and 'knowledge that' and in some instances, 'knowledge why'. They are not claiming that intelligent acts of skill do not have any thought, only that the individual has acquired the knowledge and that having habitualised it, he is able to perform it without having to think greatly about it. In the course of their duties nurses, midwives and health visitors perform many habitualised actions, eg. aseptic dressing technique, recording blood pressure, vision testing etc. When a situation arises when the habitualised knowledge is not directly applicable to the situation the actor has either to change his course of action or utilise the procedure that fits most closely the new situation. The latter course of action is fundamentally bureaucratic and not the basis of professional practice, so that it should not be encouraged. By contrast, the thoughtful professional should seek to utilise his knowledge (both 'that' and 'why') in order to respond with a new course of action. Hence, there is a sense in which theory and practice come together in an active manner when the professional practitioner has to solve a problem in the process of implementing care.

Figure 5.1 A Problem Solving Cycle

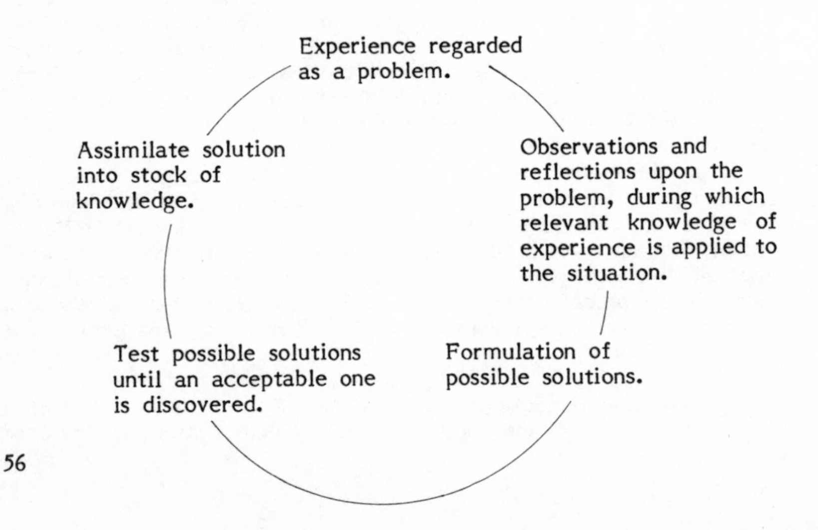

The above diagram illustrates clearly an interrelationship between theory and practice which implies that to separate them in any way would impoverish both. Ryle was clearly right in seeking to discredit the over-emphasis placed upon theory but he does not appear correct in suggesting that intelligent activity is a single act. But theory and practice are closely interrelated, so that it would be quite false to regard the teacher practitioner as 'only a teacher of skills'. She has to help the student with the combination of the two, so that she can both utilise habitualised skills and problem solving techniques as appropriate.

In precisely the same way the teacher practitioner herself needs to have a theoretical knowledge of education so that she can undertake her task as a teacher. Hence, earlier in this book the problems for the teacher practitioner, as being a member of two occupational groups, were discussed and the remainder of this chapter concentrates upon some theoretical and practical approaches to teaching.

II Teaching Styles and Models of Teaching

Non-formal teaching in individualised teaching and learning is not a stereotypical process and the teacher practitioner may adopt different approaches to the performance of her teaching role. These different approaches may be similar in many ways to those adopted by a teacher in a more formal teaching role. For instance, the teacher practitioner may be authoritarian, democratic or laissez-faire; she may regard her students as highly motivated or being inherently lazy who have to be cajoled or coerced into activity; she may see her role as implanting knowledge or in providing opportunities for her students to learn. These different approaches have usually been referred to as teaching styles but they actually reflect different approaches and models to teaching itself, so that they will be discussed here and this will lead into an explanation of the nature of teaching itself.

In the 1930's Kurt Lewin and his associates (Lippitt and White, 1958), undertook some research into different leadership styles, highlighting three approaches: authoritarian, democratic and laissez-faire. While this research was conducted with ten year old boys in group situations at youth camps and, consequently, far removed from the situation of the teacher practitioner it is mentioned here because there is a sense in which the teacher assumes a leadership role. In the teaching and learning transaction it is quite possible for the teacher practitioner to be authoritarian, democratic or even laissez-faire, although this final approach is less likely by virtue of the situation. The teacher practitioner may be authoritarian - stern, bossy, seeking always to tell and direct her student. By contrast, she may wish to do very little and let the student 'get on with it' and merely to watch her work. Lewin and his associates discovered that while the authoritarian leader appeared to get a lot of work completed as a result of a high level of activity, it only occurred during his presence since he had not really made the participants feel that the work was their own. The laissez-faire leader achieved very little, whether he was present or not. However, Lewin and his associates discovered that the democratic leader was able to achieve co-operation from the children who then worked well together on their projects whether he was present or absent from the situation, since they had decided upon what to do together and it was therefore their own work. This approach is clearly more in accord with the perspective adopted in this book and reflects the humanistic transaction between teacher practitioner and learner discussed in earlier chapters.

According to Davies (1971) the teacher is also a manager of the teaching and learning situation and McGregor (1960) highlighted two different approaches to management that have some relevance here: he called these Theory X and Theory Y. The former suggests that the manager regards the individual as having to be cajoled or coerced into activity by threat of punishment or by promise of reward because he treats the individual as fundamentally lazy. This is sometimes referred to as the "carrot-and-stick" approach. By contrast, the latter theory starts from the presupposition that the human being is self motivated and seeks to fulfil his potential. Similarity may be seen here between this management theory and the leadership research by Lewin and his associates, since Theory Y reflects a philosophy similar to that inherent in democratic leadership and is in harmony with the approach that is highlighted throughout this study, since it reflects a humanistic philosophy.

Both of the previous two processes have indicated that an ideological perspective will result in a style of leadership or management that is relevant to the teacher practitioner as she considers how to perform her role. However, these approaches have not actually been about teaching per se and it is perhaps significant to note that no simple association of philosophy and the actual style of teaching can be drawn in this manner. There are three different approaches to teaching, which are didactic, socratic and facilitative; these are both styles and categories of teaching method, and in the latter context they will form the basis for the discussion on methods. However, they are first discussed briefly here as teaching styles. Didactic teaching assumes that the teacher has knowledge to impart and that he adopts the style of 'giving out' his knowledge to the student. The socratic approach, however, assumes that the student is not an empty receptacle to be filled but rather an active thinker so that the teacher's style becomes more questioning, requiring the learner to become a problem solver and more reflective. Hence, the teacher is now seeking to draw out rather than put into the student. Facilitative teaching is a style whereby the teacher steps back from the actual learning process, having first provided the conditions in which learning can actually occur, but is available as a resource if the student requires advice or guidance.

Clearly, it may be seen that the authoritarian leader may be more likely to be a didactic teacher but the contrast may not necessarily be true. Similarly, the democratic leader is more likely to be socratic but this need not necessarily occur. Someone who holds the ideology of Theory Y may well practise all three of these teaching styles on different occasions. Hence, there is no simple association between all the styles discussed in this section even though it is easy to see some of the associations that might arise. However, from all the discussion it may be seen that there are fundamentally two models of teaching:

- a teacher-centred model, in which the teacher decides, the teacher controls and the teacher imparts knowledge
- a learner-centred model, in which the learner is involved in the decision making process in a democratic manner and the learner's acquisition of knowledge, skill and attitude is more significant than the teacher's activity.

Consequently, it may be asked - what is teaching? If teaching is not the impartation of knowledge, as is often assumed, what is it? Perhaps teaching might best be defined as the process of helping others learn. This, then, is the activity in which the teacher practitioner is involved and it is now necessary to explore some of the methods by which she might perform this activity.

III Teaching Methods for Individualised Teaching and Learning

Adults learn from experience. Perhaps that was one of the most important implications from the experiential learning cycle that was discussed earlier, so that the experience of working in the professional situation is perhaps the greatest single learning experience that can be provided for the student. Nevertheless, it is the job of the teacher practitioner to ensure that the experience provided is fully utilised and that the lessons that can be learned from it are learned efficiently and correctly, so that she needs to be competent in the use of the non-formal techniques which are applicable to the individualised teaching and learning situation. In this section six of these methods are discussed: demonstration; talk; discussion; role play and simulation; practical assignments; visits and trips. These six techniques form an approximate continuum from teacher centred to learner centred models of teaching, although in the ensuing discussion it will be seen that even the more teacher centred approaches may be utilised in a learner centred manner.

Demonstration: Demonstrating a psychomotor skill is often regarded as the method whereby the learner acquires knowledge of how to perform from an expert. Having witnessed the expert perform the learner is then expected to practise until he is as proficient as the demonstrator. This approach has been generally regarded as not having been very successful with older learners, so that according to Belbin and Belbin (1972), it has become general practice to recruit only younger people to some occupations that require manual dexterity. However, Belbin and Belbin (1972:44-45) suggest that if a skill is broken down into its component parts and that each stage is demonstrated and practised slowly and only gradually is the whole procedure unified, it is possible for older learners to acquire new skills fairly rapidly. They recognise, however, that one of the most difficult elements in this approach is that of learning each stage of the skill slowly and precisely in the first instance and only, subsequently, when the procedure is learned should it be speeded up. Following this approach, it would prove useful for teacher practitioners to analyse carefully the skills that they are required to teach and sub-divide each into discrete stages, so that in the individualised teaching and learning situation they can help the student with each of the component parts. In this way, the teacher practitioner may help the learner acquire proficiency and fluency in skills and procedures quite efficiently. This may not be as simple as it sounds since Dreyfus and Dreyfus (cited in de Tornyay and Thompson 1982:61) suggest that the expert may have incorporated the various stages of the skill into his performance so that he is unable to identify the component parts. Hence, it might be beneficial for a teacher practitioner to endeavour to undertake such an analysis whilst observing another practitioner performing that specific skill. Another factor that the teacher practitioner should consider when employing the demonstration method is whether the learner uses the same hand as herself. For instance, if the teacher practitioner is right handed and the learner left handed then she sees a different image of the practice than would her right handed colleague. Hence, if the teacher practitioner and the student work with the same hands, then the learner might be best positioned next to the teacher practitioner but, when they use opposite hands, the learner should be placed directly facing her. During demonstration the teacher practitioner should be aware of the taxonomies of objectives in the psychomotor domain discussed by Simpson and Harrow and mentioned in the third chapter of this text. However, even if the aforementioned facts are taken into consideration, a major weakness in the demonstration method is that the teacher practitioner becomes a role model and her own way of proceeding may become the approach that she teaches and expects others to perform, although it may not actually be the most effective way to perform for the student whom she is teaching.

By contrast to this approach, which is a teacher-centred method, learner-centred discovery methods of learning skills are now regarded as more efficient. Smith (1977:199) writes:

In essence, the discovery method is a style of teaching which structures a situation so that the trainee learns by activity finding out the principles and relationships himself. Thus, for example, instead of a trainee being shown a piece of equipment and given a lecture on how it works, the trainee would be given the actual piece of equipment with the parts clearly labelled. Provided that safety considerations are taken into account, the trainee learns the function of each part and how the equipment works by operating it himself.

In this approach, the teacher practitioner facilitates the learning situation and thus allows the learner to work at her own pace; she encourages the student to master the equipment as she is ready, acting as a motivator and as an aide to the reflective process. Obviously this technique can be utilised quite easily for much of the equipment that student nurses and midwives are expected to employ in a hospital and even in the community, but where there are nursing and interpersonal skills that directly involve a patient or a client this may make this particular technique inappropriate. In some instances, however, it might be possible for a student to practise skills on a dummy in a training and learning ward or even on peers, prior to practising on patients/clients, so that where this is possible the discovery method may still be used. When employing the demonstration technique, the teacher practitioner should not be too unrealistic in her expectation of the student's performance but she should seek to ensure that the latter is safe to practise before allowing her to do so when she is unsupervised. Proficient performance may take a considerable time to achieve, and the teacher practitioner should always be aware of the progress that the student makes and commend her for it, since positive feedback is always an encouragement to continue learning. However, there are skills mostly of the interpersonal kind, that may not always be learned by the discovery method and therefore more appropriate techniques should be employed.

The Talk: The talk is rather like a lecture, where the teacher practitioner addresses the student in a more formal manner and when the flow of conversation is mainly from the teacher practitioner to the student. Giving information to the student in this manner may have a place in the work of the teacher practitioner but she should be aware that this technique is generally regarded as having limited value, especially in teaching adults. Concentration spans vary and Trenaman (1951) claimed that after fifteen minutes the talk becomes an ineffective mode of communication, while Legge (1974:59) implies that for some people from four to five minutes is the maximum time that they can concentrate. However, the talk is considered a relatively easy teaching technique, so that it is frequently employed but if it is to be used by teacher practitioners then they should be aware of its limitations.

Even so, talks are often given, and frequently expected, so that it is important that teacher practitioners acquire the skills of both preparation and presentation. Talks do need careful and thorough preparation, so that the listener can follow the flow and logic of the argument. Therefore, the structure of the talk is vital, almost as important as the content, for good content has no value if the listener cannot learn it! It is wise in a short talk to have no more than two or three main points, each of which should flow logically from the other and, in addition, it is useful to have both an introduction and a conclusion. The old maxim has much validity: "First, I tells 'em what I'm going to tell 'em, then I tells 'em and then I tells 'em what I've told 'em". It is useful for listeners to know what they are about to learn, so that they can prepare their minds for it and it is beneficial to learning to help the recipient of information to pass on the crucial issues at the end. Hence, one simple structure for a talk might be:

Introduction	-	in which the rationale behind the presentation and the sequence of the main points is given
Part I	-	main body of information developed logically in a number of
Part II	-	points not necessarily
Part III	-	three
Conclusion	-	recapitulating the main points and summarising the argument.

It is always useful to prepare a talk very thoroughly and often the shorter the talk the more difficult it is to prepare because of the need to condense material, so that it may be necessary to spend longer planning a five minute address than a fifteen minute one. Many people find it very useful to write out the whole talk during preparation rather than merely sketching an outline and such thoroughness in preparation is recommended, especially in the early days of a teaching career. When the talk is prepared it may be useful to precis it for presentation purposes, e.g. using just paragraph headings on a single sheet of paper, or on postcards.

When giving a talk, even to only one student, it is necessary to ensure that, wherever possible, the physical environment is conducive to learning. For instance, the place where the talk is given should be free from constant interruption, the furniture should be comfortable and the teacher practitioner should sit in a position whereby she can maintain eye contact with the student in order to assess the extent to which the student is understanding what is being presented to her. Sheets of paper and full notes may also be a hindrance to maintaining eye contact, so that is is preferable to deliver a talk either without notes or, if this proves difficult, with as few as possible. If notes are employed, it is useful to reduce the notes to a few words about each point and, perhaps, to write each point on a postcard. In this manner the teacher practitioner will have sufficient support to give her confidence, enough material to allow her to recreate her points in her narrative and not too many notes to prevent eye contact with the student.

Even so, the limitations of this teaching technique have to be recognised and there are other methods less teacher-centred, that teacher practitioners may employ. In some instances, guided reading could replace the talk and this might be followed by a discussion.

Discussion Methods: These may appear to be a more natural approach to adopt in individualised teaching and learning than the rather stereotypical talk and there are basically three types of discussion methods that may be utilised: teacher controlled, guided and student controlled.

In teacher controlled discussion the teacher is still in charge of the interaction and she presents the topic selected for discussion, but unlike the talk, she expects some verbal participation from the student; either by responding to questions, commenting on points or issues raised and perhaps by asking the teacher questions. Nevertheless, it is the teacher who directs the discussion, controls its pace and often it is she who has selected the topic which is under consideration. Teacher practitioners may find that this technique is more realistic in the individualised teaching and learning situation in which they perform this role. As the teacher practitioner is controlling the interaction it is important that her preparation is thorough and she may well undertake similar preparation to that described for the talk, but, in addition, she may work out the points where she would like, or expect, student participation. Clearly this approach has a number of advantages over the talk including the fact that there is: student participation; active learning; less chance of the student losing concentration; opportunity for the student to disagree with the teacher; opportunity for the student to share relevant experiences; less artificiality in the non-formal teaching situation.

Guided discussion is an approach that utilises the student's experiences much more than controlled discussion. In this instance, the teacher seeks to elicit information, knowledge, ideas, etc. from the student by a carefully prepared process of questioning. This is the socratic style, which was discussed earlier in the chapter, whereby the teacher endeavours to lead the student from what she already knows into new realms of thought by building one question upon another, taking the student through a logical sequence of stages until she is able to draw conclusions or express new ideas. Because the teacher is utilising the student's knowledge and building upon her answers there could be a temptation to assume that the approach demands less preparation, but this is not so! In preparation, the teacher has to anticipate the student's response and endeavour to work out notes from those responses in order to ensure that the aims and objectives of the session are achieved. In addition, the teacher requires a sound knowledge of the subject since the student's responses may make considerable demands upon the teacher's professional expertise.

Asking questions is an art, one that the teacher practitioner should acquire in order to ensure that the learner is able to demonstrate her knowledge. Additionally, skilled questioning techniques can only enhance professional practice. Questions are asked for various reasons, eg, to obtain information, to stimulate reflection and creative thought, to assess learning outcomes, to determine learning needs, to clarify a situation, to establish and maintain social interaction. Obviously the purpose of the question will influence the way in which it is formulated and posed. Both the formulation and the manner in which it is asked will effect the response and inexperienced teacher practitioners often fail to get the type of reply that they seek from questions.

Questions may be classified in a variety of ways; de Tornyay and Thompson (1982: 65-72) categorise them as follows:

- factual or descriptive
- clarifying
- higher order
- convergent and divergent

Each of these is now briefly considered.

Factual or descriptive questions usually begin with: what; why; how; who; when; where. These questions elicit factual information which a person has memorised, a description of an event, situation, object or person. Questions of this type are:

- What factors contribute to hypothermia in the elderly?
- How is John's ulcer today?
- What foods contain calciferol?

These are the types of question that the teacher practitioner should employ to ensure that the student actually has the 'knowledge that' and if appropriate has observed accurately the client or patient.

One of the purposes of clarifying questions is to enable the learner to elaborate upon an initial response or to help her reflect upon a learning situation. This may be undertaken by:

- seeking more information and/or additional meaning
- requiring justification of a previous response
- focusing the student's attention on a related issue
- prompting
- redirecting attention

Higher order questions are more demanding than the previous types since they cannot be answered by memory recall, description or perception. These questions ask students to think and to learn from a previous experience and as such it may be seen that they are the type of questions that teacher practitioners should use to help the learner reflect upon an earlier learning experience. According to de Tornyay and Thompson (1982:68) higher order questions perform three specific functions, as the following examples show:

- evaluation, eg what were the priorities which led you to organise your caseload in this way today?
- inferences, eg what did you learn about that nursing problem as a result of caring for Mrs Smith?
- comparisons, eg What is the relationship between social class and perinatal mortality?

In contrast to the above, some questions may be posed that encourage the 'intellectually convergent' or the 'intellectually divergent' to utilise their own orientation to thinking and learning. In the convergent mode the student is encouraged to comprehend the task in hand and to focus closely upon it, whereas in the divergent approach the learner is given the opportunity to think more widely and to apply knowledge to a variety of situations in order to synthesize ideas, perceive relationships and to engage in creative problem solving.

Questions may appear threatening to students who have not been exposed to the socratic method of teaching, so that they should always be asked in a warm and friendly manner. Hence, it may be seen from the above discussion that both the type of question and the technique employed to pose it are pertinent to teaching and learning, so that it may be useful for teacher practitioners to practise this art.

Unlike the previous two approaches, student controlled discussion allows the student to ask all the questions. Obviously, the degree to which the student feels free to ask significant questions will depend upon the rapport that exists between the teacher practitioner and the student. If, for instance, the student is being continuously assessed and she feels that the teacher practitioner is her assessor rather than her teacher-guide, she may never feel able to ask such questions since she might feel that they would reveal her weaknesses rather than the strengths of an enquiring mind endeavouring to understand everything relevant to her professional practice. Hence, students should always be given the opportunity and encouraged to raise significant and searching questions both about professional practice and about the manner in which the teacher practitioner performs her dual role of teacher and professional practitioner. In other words, the teacher practitioner's professional knowledge, skills and attitudes should always be open to the student's searching enquiry. The student should be encouraged to ask questions by the teacher practitioner and the answers that she receives should always be honest. Hence, if the teacher practitioner does not know the answer to a question, she should admit to it and thus suggest that they both endeavour to discover an answer. Such an approach facilitates active learning for both the teacher practitioner and the student. But will not the teacher practitioner lose face with the student? Nobody expects the teacher practitioner to know everything, so that provided this response is not forthcoming too frequently it will do no harm to the teacher practitioner's reputation. Even so, teacher practitioners may not actually always wish to answer questions that students ask, they may wish to respond with a further question, which leads the student into further realms of knowledge. Effective teachers do not always lead students from answer to answer but often from one question to another.

While discussion methods may appear to be a little more time consuming, they are approaches which the teacher practitioner might wish to adopt since they allow her to be sure that the student has actually learned the knowledge and that she is also able to express what she knows. Additionally, the guided discussion technique is useful to help students reflect upon their learning experiences, enabling them to capitalise upon their learning and to pursue more thoroughly the ideas that the experiences set in motion. Hence, they are beneficial techniques to be employed in individualised teaching and learning.

Role Play and Simulation: These teaching and learning methods are basically the dramatization of 'real life' events in which the role players enact the roles which either they themselves, or others, would perform in the actual situation. The primary purpose is to enable the learners to experience in a more protected environment the emotions and the problems of people in everyday living. Clearly it has a number of uses in professional education, some of which will be referred to below. Role play is frequently unscripted but carefully prepared before the event, whereas simulation is the creation of an actual situation in which the procedures are far less spontaneous and are often played out over a longer period of time than role play. Hence, simulation is perhaps a less useful method to the teacher practitioner than role play.

There are many advantages in using these techniques because not only do they involve the student in active learning but that learning is of an affective nature in which it is important for practitioners to consider their interpersonal skills, often in very stressful situations. This approach to their preparation, therefore, enables them to focus upon quite specific incidents and skills. Role play can be employed to help a student experience a specific role prior to her having to perform it professionally, to help the student to consider the attitudes and feelings that surface on such occasions and to enable her to analyse and practise the social skills necessary in the professional situation. Despite these advantages, this technique does not appear to be used as frequently as it might, which may be because acting and playing may be considered to be childish or only adult if they occur in the right place, like a theatre. Additionally, it may also not be used because it appears artificial and the actors feel inhibited or because it is recognised that such dramatic interaction might provoke an emotional situation that the teacher does not feel confident enough to handle.

To some extent the sense of artificiality can be overcome in the work of the teacher practitioner if she explains to the student that role play is a teaching and learning method that provides a safe situation for the student to work out her role performance in a new situation, to enact a difficult situation, and to aid reflection upon a previously problematic experience. During the initial preparation for the role play the teacher practitioner should explain the rationale behind the session and give precise details of the ideas and roles that she and the student are going to perform. She should also indicate that both participants are free to stop the role play at any time but whenever they complete it there will be a period afterwards during which they can discuss quietly the situation that has been enacted, the process through which they have gone and the emotions that they have experienced. Like all effective teaching techniques, this one demands very careful planning by the teacher practitioner, the more so in this instance because the emotions and attitudes of individuals may be displayed in a more open manner than is considered natural and normal in contemporary society. The usefulness of the approach may be seen in the way that it incorporates actual professional situations into the teaching and learning situation. Many examples could be given but two only will be provided here. Consider the distressing situation of a health visitor going to a young mother who had, on the previous evening, found her three month old son dead in his cot; the student could play the health visitor and the teacher practitioner play the mother. Another situation might be that of the district nurse visiting a patient who has carcinoma of the lung and who suspects her condition, although she has never been informed of it by her doctor. The patient asks the district nurse if she has cancer: the student might play the role of the district nurse and the teacher practitioner that of the patient. These examples are possible situations in professional practice and they are provided only to illustrate the use of this technique in the preparation of professionals. In some role play it might be useful for the student to play the role of the patient in order to gain empathy and to understand more about her own professional role.

Some teacher practitioners may not feel confident in the use of this technique and they may, therefore, seek to avoid using it. However, it has considerable use in professional training so that it is a technique with which they should be familiar, and which they should consider employing. However, it should be used with caution because it can create emotional release, so that it might be wise for the teacher practitioner to participate in role playing exercises before she introduces it into her own teaching.

Student Assignments: The practical assignment is one in which the teacher encourages the student to undertake a piece of work on her own; it may be written, research orientated or skill based and it may be teacher directed or student initiated. In some training courses where it is considered that the theory is taught by one teacher and the practice is taught by someone in the clinical work situation, there is a tendency for the latter not to be expected to be involved in setting assignments or work for the student. However, motivating a student to undertake an assignment is a method of facilitating the student's learning and should be encouraged so long as the student is given sufficient time to undertake the task and that it does not interfere with the assessment procedure of the course which has been approved by the statutory body. Such an activity may arise from: a controlled discussion session; from articles; from suggestions by the teacher practitioner that the student should find out about a specific procedure or practice; from a much more didactic talk after which the teacher practitioner suggests that the student should read a number of articles on a specific topic and make a synopsis of them; from a demonstration of skill, after which the student is asked to practise it until it has been mastered, etc. However, it is also possible for assignments to precede a teaching session where, for instance, the teacher practitioner might explain to a student that in a few days time she will be given a specific role or responsibility and that she should discover what is entailed; the teacher practitioner might then plan a socratic guided discussion a few days later in anticipation that the student would have already acquired some knowledge about it. Thus it may be seen that not all assignments have to be assessed course work but that a variety of assignments may be used, often in conjunction with other teaching methods, by the teacher practitioner.

Visits and Trips: The teacher practitioner may also be a facilitator of the student's learning by providing opportunity for the latter to have a learning need met outside of the actual professional practice situation in which she performs. This may be undertaken on the basis that she understands the student's learning need and is aware of other people who, or situations which, might be able to help the student satisfy that need effectively. She may, for instance, arrange for a student to visit a centre of excellence, an expert in a discipline or skill, a colleague who has within her professional practice and care patients whose physical or social condition is such that the student should have knowledge and expertise. Finally, the teacher practitioner may arrange for the student to visit other students so that they can exchange information and ideas.

When visits and trips are arranged, it is necessary for the teacher practitioner to make careful arrangements, using the appropriate official channels in order to ensure that the relevant personnel are aware of what has been arranged and the purpose of the student's visit. The teacher practitioner should also prepare the student prior to the visit, so that she is enabled to obtain maximum benefit from the experience. Additionally, the teacher practitioner should ensure that after such a visit she conducts a follow-up session in order to assist the student to crystallise her ideas from the learning experience that has been provided. Finally, the teacher practitioner must ensure that the normal after-visit courtesies are undertaken by both herself and the student, so that the person who received the visitors is aware of its usefulness and that it has been appreciated.

It may be seen from the above discussions that a combination of teaching methods may be more useful than employing only one technique per topic. A variety of approaches may enrich the learning experience, so that the more proficient the teacher practitioner is in utilising different techniques the more efficiently will the student be prepared to perform her professional role. Since the teacher practitioner may be a facilitator of the student's learning rather than merely a provider of information and instructor of skills for the student to learn, she may not only teach the student all that she knows but she may actually teach the student more than she knows and that can only be enriching for the profession as a whole and for the patients and clients whom the student will serve when she is qualified.

IV Some Other Teaching Methods

The teacher practitioner is sometimes invited to give a presentation before a group of people, eg students in a college or school of nursing, clients in a health centre, so that she should be aware of some of the techniques of teaching groups but since this is not her main teaching role less emphasis is placed upon it here. Even so, some reference is made to some of the main approaches that she may wish to employ although if she is particularly interested in this she might be wise to read some of the texts recommended in the selection of further reading at the end of this book. The two main methods mentioned here, the lecture and discussion methods, have a number of variations although the same dichotomy of teacher centred and learner centred approaches is appropriate.

The Lecture: This is the normal approach expected from a visiting speaker since she has some knowledge and information that she is expected to convey to the learners within a specfied time. However, there are a number of variations on the lecture, including: the normal straight lecture, the lecture followed by discussion and the lecture interspersed with discussion. Each of these are now examined briefly.

The normal lecture technique is perhaps the most common form of teaching and yet despite its popularity many criticisms have been levelled at it, so that it is important to put this method into perspective. Bligh (1971:4) summarises research on the topic when he argues that:

> (1) with the exception of programmed learning the lecture is as effective as any other method of transmitting information, but not more effective; (2) most lectures are not as effective as more active methods for the production of thought; and (3) changing student attitudes should not normally be the major objective of the lecture.

Thus it may be seen that only in the transmission of information is the lecture as effective as other methods of teaching, but it must also be recognised that much of the research that led to this conclusion was not actually conducted with adult students, although Trenaman's research on the length of time that people will listen to radio broadcasts was, in fact, with adults (see Legge 1974).

If the teacher practitioner is invited to give a lecture she may feel duty-bound to concur with the request and use the method, since this will also be what the audience expect from her. If she delivers a lecture, there are a number of points relevant to her preparation discussed in the earlier section on the 'Talk'. In addition a number of common errors that she should try to avoid are listed below:

- Preparing too much material. The conscientious lecturer may prepare far too much material and as she is making the presentation she might realise that she has not sufficient time to deliver it all, consequently she tries to speed up her presentation and, by so doing, she loses the learners' concentration.
- Speaking for too long. As Trenaman showed, concentration spans vary from about five to about twenty minutes, so that there tends to be a lessening of concentration after the first few minutes and this may result in much of the material presented being lost to her hearers.
- Being bound to notes. The teacher practitioner should try to avoid being bound to notes since she will, otherwise, lose eye contact with her listeners and, therefore, be less sensitive to their expressed needs. If the volume of notes is reduced, then there is more likely to be a genuine interchange between speaker and learners.
- Speaking with one's back to the audience. This occurs most frequently if the speaker is using a blackboard and it often results in adults, especially those with slightly impaired hearing, losing some of the words uttered by the speaker. If the lecturer wants to use the blackboard it is worth remaining silent whilst writing, although an alternative approach would be to employ an overhead projector.
- Walking around the room while speaking. This may also result in the hard of hearing finding it difficult to follow

every word that the lecturer speaks. Even so, this is not to suggest the the lecturer should remain immobile during the delivery, only that the teacher practitioner is aware of the potential problem.

- Not speaking loudly enough. This is a common occurrence with inexperienced lecturers and it may be useful for the teacher practitioner to pick out a member of the audience who is rather close to the back of the room and imagine that she is addressing that one individual, although she should not focus solely upon that person, since this might cause embarrassment.
- Speaking too quickly. Often a speaker tries to ensure everybody hears by merely trying to speak more loudly but it is also most beneficial for her to slow down the speed of her presentation and to ensure that the ends of the words are clearly pronounced.

Whilst the lecture has a number of limitations, some of which may be partially overcome by variations upon the technique, the fact that it is a teacher centred approach must also be recognised.

The lecture-discussion is an approach quite frequently expected of visiting lecturers, although the concluding discussion often tends to take the form of questions being raised by members of the audience and addressed to the speaker, usually seeking clarification and amplification of a point raised in the presentation itself. However, this technique may take the form of a short presentation by the speaker followed by group discussion with, or without, a concluding plenary session. If the teacher practitioner wishes to employ this approach she should ensure that the institution inviting her is prepared for the use of the methods, that the room is suitable and that the chairs are not fixed together. If this technique is used, the teacher practitioner should prepare carefully the question(s) that the groups are to discuss and ensure that they are directly related to some issue(s) raised in the initial address. Where small groups are used in this way, the teacher practitioner should ensure that all the group members know each other and if they do not, she should tell them to introduce themselves to each other at the outset. If there is to be a plenary session during which the conclusions of each group are to be reported, the teacher practitioner should ensure that a rapporteur is elected from each group, and, if necessary, that there is a group secretary and chairman. However, if the time is limited she may wish to delegate these roles in a more arbitrary manner.

When presentation and discussion are interspersed it is much harder for the lecturer to form small groups and move chairs, etc. so that the teacher practitioner may wish to ask questions and pose problems to the listeners at pre-selected times in her address. This is a useful approach and it does help overcome the problem of lapsed concentration. However, if the room in which the teacher practitioner is speaking is arranged with chairs in rows she is unlikely to generate much group discussion because there is little or no eye contact between the listeners, so that all the response will be directed to her. If, on the other hand, the chairs are so arranged to allow participants to see each other, then the teacher practitioner may manage to get interaction between the group as a result of her questions. This may be less likely with a large audience and in this instance responses to the teacher practitioner's questions may be dominated by the less retiring members of the audience. This approach does allow the lecturer to plan her time carefully, even though she may be forced to intervene in a discussion in order to pursue the goals of the session, if she so desires. However, if there is good and valid discussion she may not wish to follow her preconceived plan.

Discussion Methods: It will already have been recognised how important discussion methods are to the teaching of adults. There are two other approaches that are referred to here even though they have similarities to the above techniques. Bligh (1971:126) mentions the use of free-group discussion, which he defines as a learning situation in which the topic and the direction are controlled by the student group. While this is a useful method for a teacher, it is not necessarily one that the teacher practitioner is likely to employ when she is invited to speak at a local college or school of nursing. By contrast, she might well employ a problem centred discussion technique, where she sets groups problems to solve prior to her entering the discussion with the students. This approach does encourage analytical thinking, ability to make decisions, and the opportunity to evaluate them. It is a useful method for the teacher practitioner to employ in a situation where she is able to have a longer time with the learners.

Having examined a number of different teaching methods that the teacher practitioner might find useful in the course of her work, it is now necessary to consider the use of teaching aids.

V Teaching Aids

Teaching aids are used most frequently in a more formal classroom setting but they are also useful in non-formal teaching and learning. The purpose of this section is to examine briefly some of the aids that might be useful to the teacher practitioner but not to refer to the wider variety of audio-visual aids that may be employed in the classroom. Four groups of aids are discussed here: audio-cassettes, charts, handouts and models.

Audio-cassettes: At the present moment there are few audio-cassettes available for purchase that would be useful for the work of the teacher practitioner. Nevertheless, this does not prevent her preparing her own and this would be especially useful for the teacher practitioner whose work is located in the community and who is, therefore, expected to use a car. In many instances students also have their own cars and thus, it is quite possible for the teacher practitioner to prepare her own cassettes and to loan them to a student when she is visiting independently from the teacher practitioner. Subjects that might be covered, include: helping prepare the student for a difficult visit; helping the student assess the visit by raising a series of questions which she should consider in assessing her practice; a socratic-type exercise to follow a teaching and learning session in which they have both been engaged; an exercise to consider an article in a journal in a critical manner, etc. The use of the audio-cassette is both time saving and an approach that helps the student create a habit of independent learning. This method may also be useful in a hospital setting where the teacher practitioner could prepare a number of cassettes about specific relevant aspects of practice which the student could use when an appropriate time arose, eg. describing a specific procedure or raising questions about it. (The student should be advised to ensure that audio cassette recorders are kept in a safe place.)

Both in the community and hospital settings the use of this technique depends upon the availability of resources and the willingness of teacher practitioners to employ less common approaches to teaching. It might also be possible for the teacher practitioner to use the technical staff in schools of nursing and colleges to help her prepare such cassettes.

Charts and Diagrams: Some people learn better through visual perception than they do by hearing, so that it is useful for the teacher practitioner to prepare or collect her own library of charts and diagrams. These may refer to any aspect of theory or practice. While a local college department or school of nursing may have its own resource centre which the teacher practitioner may use, she may discover that she needs visual aids that relate specifically to the type of work which she is undertaking and those with a directly practical orientation, so that it may be better if she obtained, prepared and stored for herself. Hence, she may have to prepare her own and having done so for a specific occasion she may wish to keep it for future use. Not all visual aids have to be made by the teacher practitioner and many charts and diagrams are produced by commercial companies, especially in order to advertise their own products. These are often supplied freely, or may be obtained inexpensively, so that it is useful for teacher practitioners to be aware of these sources of visual information and to collect as much relevant material as possible. These are often mentioned in the nursing press and may be purchased from such organisations as the Health Education Council. Having collected a library of charts and diagrams it is necessary to have a storage facility, such as a cupboard or a filing cabinet, which is readily available to the teacher practitioner. But once material is stored there are a number of points that should be borne in mind by the teacher practitioner when she uses it on a later occasion, including:

- whether it is still accurate and up-to-date
- whether it is completely relevant to the individualised teaching and learning situation for which she intends to use it
- whether it is appropriate to make the points that the teacher practitioner wishes it to make in the specific situation

Handout: The handout is a useful teaching aid since many students find that they learn best by reading about the subject and reflecting upon it, either before or after a teaching session, so that the teacher practitioner may wish to give a student a handout prior to a session with an agreement to discuss it on a specific forthcoming day or she may provide a handout after a session for the student to study. Most handouts have to be prepared by the teacher practitioner and initially this may be a time consuming process, but once a handout is prepared and copies of it made then it can be used on subsequent occasions. Handouts do not have to be typed but they should be neatly prepared. Photographs and diagrams can be included in a handout, if appropriate, provided that they can be photocopied.

Another type of a handout that the teacher practitioner may find useful is prepared reading material, such as an article in a journal, a research report or a chapter of a book, or even a list of references. Having directed a student to such material or loaned a copy to the student, it is essential for the teacher practitioner to conduct a socratic style teaching and learning session about it at a later date in order to ensure that the student has critically understood the material provided.

Models: Many schools of nursing and college departments have models relevant to many aspects of the course of study in their resource centres to which students often have ready access. Occasionally, however, a teacher practitioner may desire to use models in relation to the work that she is undertaking with a student. If she has access to the resource centre, or museum, then it is useful for her to have borrowing rights for equipment, but if there is no such centre or she does not have ready access to it then she may wish to construct her own models. This need not be an expensive undertaking since many models can be constructed from materials that might normally be thrown away as useless. Such a task is time consuming but it will be rewarding if the end product is enriched learning by the student, as fieldwork and practical work teachers who have prepared such material have discovered.

It will be noted from a number of references in this section that teacher practitioners may wish to store the material that they collect or prepare. Hence, they may wish to prepare their own small resource centres. Additionally, they should be aware of places where they can acquire teaching aids such as a resource centre in schools of nursing, local college centres, libraries, the local Health Education Department, national resource centres etc.

VI Preparing a Teaching and Learning Session

It will have become clear from the foregoing discussion that in order to ensure that a teaching and learning session has a good chance of success it is necessary for the teacher practitioner to undertake considerable preparation, so that it is now important to focus upon this process. Basically a number of elements have to be considered and these include: the aims and objectives of the session, content, method, location, timing and evaluation. Each of these points is discussed in turn.

Aims and Objectives: Since the aims of a course usually reflect its broad philosophical intentions, they are of less significance to the teacher practitioner's immediate preparation than are the course objectives. Even so, the teacher practitioner should have agreed with the student the aims of the practical professional experience which is being provided. These should reflect the overall aims of the course and since these do not usually vary from one session to the next, it is the objectives of the teaching session that should be the immediate concern of the teacher practitioner's preparation. Clearly these also need to be in accord with the previously formulated aims.

It will be recalled that certain reservations were raised about behavioural objectives in the third chapter mostly because learning is much wider than behaviour, so that it might be wiser for a teacher practitioner to formulate the objectives in non-behavioural terms, unless there is agreement between her and the student in respect of a specific skill or procedure. In this instance they may wish to agree upon specific behavioural objectives. Naturally, the teacher practitioner should discuss with the student the programme of events for two or three days in advance in order that they might agree upon objectives for specific sessions. Objectives should have a degree of specificity and be the guidelines for the teacher practitioner in preparing individual teaching and learning programmes.

Some schools of nursing and colleges provide specific objectives for the various designated clinical areas and those responsible for the teaching and learning in these locations are expected to use these. Usually they have been developed by various grades of staff together. If teacher practitioners or the students are dissatisfied with any of the objectives with which they are presented they should discuss these with the personnel who provided them, so that amendments might be made to ensure that they are relevant to the situation.

Content: Having prepared the objectives the teacher practitioner may then select relevant content matter and order it in a logical sequence, so that it starts from the point at which the previous session had concluded, or from a point about which the teacher practitioner knows the student is already knowledgeable, or from a relevant situation. The progression of the content should be carefully prepared even though the sequence may not be retained during the teaching and learning session because of interventions from the student. Many teachers feel more confident, especially early in their careers, if they have actually written out the content in full prior to teaching it and it is a form of preparation to be recommended, even though in the non-formal teaching and learning situation full notes may not actually be employed. When a teacher practitioner is not perfectly sure of the content herself she should consult a relevant authority (book or person) prior to teaching so that she does not knowingly provide the student with incorrect information.

Methods: At the same time as the teacher practitioner is selecting the content she should also be planning the method(s) that she is going to employ and these should be built into her lesson plan. Consideration should be given to a number of factors when selecting the method, including:

- the student's preferred learning style
- the approaches the teacher practitioner would prefer to employ
- the way that the selected content might best be presented
- which teaching aids would enhance the teaching and learning session
- the location which is available for the session

Location and Timing: If the teacher practitioner has a choice of locations for the teaching and learning session, then deciding upon which location to use is an important element in its preparation. It is also important to recognise that in planning the location, consideration will also need to be given to the seating arrangements to ensure eye contact, whether the session should take place over a cup of coffee, etc. The session should also be kept to the planned length so that it does not interfere into any of the other professional commitments of either participant.

Evaluation: After any teaching and learning process the teacher practitioner should evaluate what has been undertaken. Evaluation is not merely asking whether the objectives of the session have been achieved but whether all aspects of the teaching and learning session had been satisfactory. Included in the questions that the teacher practitioner should ask, are:

- Did the objectives reflect the overall aims of the course?
- Were the objectives achieved?
  If not, why not? If so, why?
- Were the objectives satisfactory?
  If not, why not?
- Was the content sufficient?
  If not, why not?
- Was the content relevant?

If not, why not?

- Was the presentation of the content structured in a logical manner?
  If not, were there justifiable reasons why this occurred?
- Were the methods employed the most effective?
  Which other approaches might have been utilised effectively?
- Was the time and/or place of the session appropriate?
  If not, when and/or where else might it have been conducted?
- Was the relationship between teacher practitioner and student harmonious?
  How else might they have been improved?
- How else might the teaching and learning session have been improved?

At the end of such an evaluation the teacher practitioner should be in a position to determine the strengths and the weaknesses of the teaching and learning session that she has conducted. Evaluation is a matter of both knowing the strengths and the weaknesses of a session. It is as important for the teacher practitioner to be aware of her strengths as it is for her to know her weaknesses, so that she can continue to improve her own performance.

Occasionally, such an evaluation session might be conducted jointly by the teacher practitioner and the student so that the former has another perception of her performance. The extent to which the student should be involved will depend upon the relationship between the two, but it would be quite out of keeping with the ideals of education if it were not to occur.

Conclusion

This chapter has examined the teaching role of the teacher practitioner, a role that is significant to the preparation of new recruits to a profession. However, the majority of teacher practitioners also perform another significant role during this period of preparation, that of assessor, so that the next chapter explores the nature of assessment.

Chapter Six

ASSESSING STUDENTS

Not only does the teacher practitioner teach the student, she is frequently required to act as the student's assessor, which in some instances entails reporting on the student's suitability for admission to the profession. The responsibility for making such comments is one that is not assumed lightly by teacher practitioners and an aspect of the role that some do not like to perform. This reluctance is perfectly understandable since the teacher practitioner's report may, in some circumstances adversely affect a student's career and even prevent the individual actually entering the profession. Nevertheless, its performance is an element of the same responsibilty that she has to the patients/clients, that of ensuring that they are always rendered the best possible service.

This chapter focuses upon the subject of assessment and has six main sections. The first explores the nature of assessment and this is followed by a rationale for assessing students, different types of assessment are discussed in the third section while the next considers some useful techniques in undertaking the process, the fifth examines self and peer assessment and the final section suggests that one of the main elements of the teacher practitioner's role is that of teaching the art of self-assessment.

1 The Nature of Assessment

Assessment is a normal part of any social interaction. Whenever a person is introduced to another individual and thereafter spends some time in social intercourse with that individual, there is likely to occur a reflective comment on either the nature of the person or of the social interaction, eg 'he was a nice fellow', or 'she is really quite remarkable', or 'that conversation was enjoyable'. These comments are the essence of assessment: that they are evaluating a person, an interaction or a situation. The assessor places a value upon something that, for him, did not necessarily have one before. In the case of the first two examples given here, the value is that which one person places upon another, ie, nice or remarkable. Other people may, or may not, agree with the assessment since it is quite subjective.

Yet the teacher practitioner's assessment of the student should not be quite as subjective as this, or else entry to the profession would be rather a precarious business. However, in other branches of education and in other forms of examination, such as the written essay type examination, it is recognised that subjectivity plays a significant part in assessment. Even very experienced examiners can differ by a considerable amount when marking the same essay (see, for example, Jarvis, 1978), so that even written examinations have been designed using other techniques in order to make them more objective, eg, multiple choice questions. However, whilst some approaches may be useful, they are not without their problems. Since subjectivity is recognised as being part of the assessment process, it should not cause the teacher practitioner undue stress, unless it is directed towards or against a person rather than her practice, a point that will be discussed in the fourth part of this chapter. In practical work assessments many attempts have been made to ensure that there is some objectivity and many schools or nursing and departments in colleges, etc. have issued checklists of skills/procedures that should be taught and assessed during practice. These lists may provide useful guidelines but they do not eradicate the element of subjectivity because the teacher practitioner must still be satisfied with the way by which the student performs the requisite skill/procedure and also her approach to the overall well-being of patient or client.

Hence, it may be concluded that the satisfaction will be related to the teacher practitioner's own expectations of how that skill etc. should be performed. This should be the case whether, or not, she is working to a checklist, undertaking a ward-based assessment, working in a continuous assessment situation or working with the student in a normal professional practice situation. Thus the standard that the teacher practitioner utilises in the assessment of students might well be related to those that are exhibited in her own professional practice and these should be the rigorous standards of the highly professional practitioner.

It might well be asked whether all assessment is subjective in this manner and the response must clearly depend upon the nature of the knowledge, skill or attitude being assessed. Certain forms of knowledge are indisputable, eg, the specifications of a law or the precise dosages of a certain drug, so that the student is either correct or incorrect when stating this. In these instances the teacher practitioner is able to specify quite objectively that the student either does not does not know specific legislation or certain drug dosages. But in many other instances no such possibilities exist since there may, for instance, be a variety of ways of undertaking a task or implementing a procedure and a multitude of different approaches to a patient/client. In these cases, the teacher practitioner may wish to be objective in stating that a student implemented a procedure in a specific manner or interacted with a patient/client in a certain way and that in the outcome the procedure was completed or that the interaction resulted in specific information being transmitted to the patient/client. Rowntree (1977:6) calls this descriptive assessment. But the teacher practitioner is also expected to make a judgment on the practice or interaction and it is at this point that the subjectivity enters. She may wish to specify that the student implemented the procedure in a manner other than that which she herself would employ but that the implementation and its outcome were efficient and satisfactory. Here the assessment is a combination of the descriptive and the judgmental and it is in the latter that the teacher practitioner's own standards are important.

It will be noted immediately that this form of assessment, like some forms of teaching, is teacher centred but later in this chapter reference will be made to some learner centred methods of assessment. Before this is undertaken, however, it is necessary to explore the rationale for assessment.

II Rationale for Assessment

Earlier in the book it was argued that at the heart of the teaching and learning process there is a diagnostic function, in which the teacher and the learner actually assess together the strengths and weaknesses of the student in order to plan her future learning experiences. This diagnostic appraisal, which may also be called formative assessment, is self-evidently fundamental to individualised teaching and learning. It is something that does not only occur at the outset of the student's professional practical experience but it should be a continuing process throughout the whole period, so that the learning experiences provided for the student may be most relevant for her. By undertaking this activity the teacher practitioner and the student gain feedback about the latter's learning and about her future learning needs, whereas the former also gains similar information and also she is able to assess the efficiency of her own teaching methods, etc. In addition to providing feedback to both participants, it should also help motivate the student to continue to learn in order to satisfy both herself and the teacher practitioner of her ability. These three factors are teaching and learning orientated and in the first instance they are the most significant reasons for undertaking such a process, even though they may not be the most commonly assumed reasons why assessment is necessary.

Perhaps the most common reason given for assessment is that of the maintenance of standards. Obviously any profession must ensure that new recruits to its ranks have, prior to entry, achieved professionally accepted standards. This is the prime responsibility that the profession has to its clients/patients in order to provide the best service and, thereby, maintain public trust and support. While both health visiting and district nursing delegate the total responsibility of assessing the knowledge, skills and attitudes of new recruits to the local teaching centres, this is not so true of all other branches of nursing and midwifery. Yet in all instances, much of the responsibility of both preparing the student in the professional practice situation and assessing her in it rests with the teacher practitioner. It is the teacher practitioner, as a result of her own experience and education, who may recommend that a learner should be accepted into the profession either, because she has achieved standards acceptable to herself as the experienced professional who has been given that responsibility by the profession or because the learner is improving and should achieve those standards before she enters the practice. In this latter instance it is important that the teacher practitioner should expect high standards from her students and that in order to achieve them she should maintain high standards herself. To expect high standards is important since it ensures that those whom the teacher practitioner recommends for entry to the profession have achieved, or are in the process of achieving, a level of competency in practice that should stand them in good stead when they become fully fledged members to the profession.

III Types of Assessment

It has, perhaps, become quite evident that there are a number of different types of assessment and that three have already been mentioned:

- formative: diagnostic and occuring during the teaching and learning programme
- summative: a final assessement that occurs at the end of a course, an examination
- continuing or continuous: in which assessment is regarded as an on-going process thoughout the course

Nursing also has its four specified practical clinical assessments which may be regarded as summative, even though these may not actually occur at the end of the course, since once an assessment has been completed successfully there is no need for it to be repeated.

In some areas continuous assessment is more popular and as it is in accordance with the demands of diagnostic appraisal it obviously has its merits since it might continue to form the basis of the teaching and learning programme. It is also a method that has considerable popularity among some nurses (Spruce, 1983) even though it is not without its drawbacks, such as continued stress and potential interference in the relationship between the teacher practitioner and the learner. Individual summative assessments, eg. oral examinations, ward-based assessments, may be short, sharp and painful when they occur but for some students continuous assessment may be long, drawn-out and nagging. Hence, not all students view continuous assessment as beneficial. Obviously the degree of stress does depend upon the relationship between the teacher practitioner and the learner since if there is a harmonious relationship between them the latter will be aware of how she is progressing and, provided that her progress is satisfactory, she should be able to enjoy her practice with few fears. However, this may not always be the case with the weaker student who may fear failure. She may be worried about the teacher practitioner's role as assessor, in the same way that some fear the supervisor's appraisal function, and this may result in her not asking questions, discussing her problems, etc since she will be afraid that she is revealing her weaknesses to her assessor. In these instances, therefore, the role of assessor may interfere with both the relationship and the teacher practitioner's teaching role because the learner's presentation of herself is slightly false or overconfident. When this occurs a great deal of responsibility lies with the teacher practitioner to overcome this specific problem and her own sensitivity and social skills are important if she is to be able to help the student use her time as a learner most efficiently.

When continuous assessment is introduced into a long course, eg. the three year course of general nurse training, it is very rare for the learner to have the same teacher practitioner and assessor thoughout, so that while the assessment may be continuous in one sense it is inevitably discontinuous in another. Teacher practitioners and assessors have different standards and expect different responses from students, so that different parts of the course might be more difficult than others, etc. Additionally, the records that one teacher practitioner or assessor makes may be passed on to another, so that the second teacher practitioner or assessor may be influenced by the judgments of the first, and a self-fulfilling prophecy created. These are not light problems. However, the main reasons for raising them here are to emphasize the discontinuous nature of continuous assessment and the problem of being so influenced by the previous report so that the student is not actually being assessed independently but seen through the eyes of a previous teacher practitioner or assessor.

Throughout this text considerable emphasis has been placed upon the student assessing her own strengths and weaknesses and discussing them with the teacher practitioner, so that it must be recognised that not all assessment is necessarily teacher-centred. There is also student-centred assessment. Two forms of student-centred assessment, peer and self assessment, are discussed later in this chapter. Obviously self assessment is an important element in the type of teaching and learning transaction that has been discussed here in which both teacher practitioner and learner collaborate in the formative assessment procedure. Heron (1981) recognises the significance of this type of assessment, which he calls collaborative assessment and while this is at the heart of the individualised teaching and learning transaction, it would be quite false if something of the same form were not to occur at the summative stage. Ultimately the responsibility at that stage is the teacher practitioner's but the collaborative enterprise may be more accurate in the long term and it may remove some of the fear of the assessor's role that some weaker students have, so that it would be recommended here that even in the final summative assessment the same philosophy should prevail in as far as it is possible. Clearly, the teacher practitioner may occasionally have the very unpleasant task of recommending that a student be deferred but, in this case, the earlier collaboration should even make this activity a little easier since the student will be aware of the teacher practitioner's own standards.

IV Techniques in Assessment

It will be clearly recognised by now that the teacher practitioner's role must entail that she is an assessor as well as a teacher and that any complete division between the two functions would be artificial. In order to teach, the teacher practitioner must be an assessor and assessment should precede as well as follow teaching. Hence, it is important that the teacher practitioner is familiar with the techniques of assessment. Initially, there are a number of basic requisites that the teacher practitioner should undertake:

- look: the teacher practitioner should always be most observant when she has a student working with her. Such observation need not be formal nor need it be overt; the teacher practitioner should, however, always be aware of the learner's actions and when the time is more appropriate she may wish to use her observation as one of the resources for her teaching.
- listen: to what the student says both to her and to others who are in their company. Often what the student expresses overall will convey to the teacher practitioner both some of the student's learning needs and her attitudes.
- listen: to what others say about the student. Patients, colleagues and others may all comment to the teacher practitioner.
  Clearly the patient's/client's observations are important, not because he/she knows the technicalities of professional practice but because he/she is the recipient of the service and this is as important as any other observation made. Colleagues may also comment and these should also be listened to with great care. However, the morality of asking for comments from other people is questionable, unless it has first been discussed with the student.
- discuss: with the student what she has seen or heard. This discussion is part of the diagnostic process that should be a continuous element in the teaching and learning transaction.

- decide: ultimately a conclusion has to be reached and this should be as a result of discussion. However, if an assessor is in doubt, it is always professional to take a second opinion, even though the first assessor may not appear to know her own mind. Even so, this should not be used as a method of abrogating the teacher practitioner's own responsibility.

Having highlighted the above process, it is also important to examine some of the more specific elements in the assessment procedure and these aspects will be focused upon here: the traditional ward-based assessment and the checklist type of approach that is sometimes used in the community and continuous assessment.

In the traditional ward-based assessments, the learner informs the ward sister or clinical teacher if she is a "recognised" National Board assessor when she is ready to undertake her assessment and then the necessary arrangements are made. However, this is the creation of an artificial situation but the assessor should do everything in her power to ensure that the artificiality is minimal. Hence, the assessor's behaviour should be no more formal than it is usually, she should endeavour to ensure that everything in the clinical situation is as normal as possible and that the whole procedure occurs in as natural a setting as it would in normal professional practice. The assessor should ensure that the learner is put at her ease beforehand but be aware that by trying too hard to free the learner of any anxiety she may actually exacerbate the situation. Hence, even the process of putting the student at her ease should be carefully performed and perhaps this is best done in the days and weeks before the actual assessment occurs by ensuring that the technique or the management process is practised to such a high standard that the student is confident of her own ability to undertake the necessary requirements. No learner should be expected to undertake an assessment unless that confidence exists and herein lies an important role for the teacher practitioner. She should prepare the learner to pass the assessment and expect her to do so. Belbin and Belbin (1972:167-168) note that it does not help the student to feel that if she fails she can always try again. In addition they record the technique adopted by the driving instructor with the most successful record of teaching older persons to drive London Transport buses who claimed that he never mentioned failure and he always acted as if he knew that they were going to pass. By contrast, one with a far higher failure rate claimed that he could spot someone who was going to fail very early in the teaching and learning process. Hence, the teacher practitioner should prepare the student to pass the assessment.

If the teacher practitioner is also the assessor it is an interesting question to note how the expectations that she has as teacher practitioner may influence her opinions as assessor. If the student who performs the technique or procedure well in normal ward practice does not do so well during the formal assessment, should she pass? Likewise, should a student who performs better during the assessment than she does in normal ward practice be given the benefit of any doubt that the assessor may have? Clearly this has not a simple solution and yet it is a realistic problem since examinations of all types should be fair, replicable and relevant to professional practice (Jarvis 1983a: 106-109).

Often in the community the teacher practitioner has a checklist of procedures and skills that she is expected to ensure that the student has performed successfully whilst gaining professional fieldwork experience, but it might be more beneficial if the teacher practitioner used the checklist with the student diagnostically, so that they could consider the list early in the practice and then plan the teaching and learning sessions in relation to the student's perceived learning needs. In this way the checklist becomes the focus of tutorial sessions between the teacher practitioner and the student and a basis of planning teaching and learning. Hence, it can enrich the process of professional preparation, whereas failure to discuss it might result in impoverished teaching and learning and an incomplete survey of the total demands of practice because of the type of caseload with which the teacher practitioner is working at the time of the professional practical experience.

In continuous assessment the diagnostic process should continue throughout the period of professional practice but it will be very important for the teacher practitioner to maintain a very full record of the process so that she can ensure that the whole area of professional practice is covered by one means or another and so that she can monitor carefully all aspects of the student's progress. It is perhaps most significant that the teacher practitioner should maintain such a record so that at the end of the practice she is able to write a full report about the student, but even more important is that through monitoring the student's progress in all aspects of professional practice she is not merely able to report on the student but she is in a position to offer a prognosis on the likelihood of the student's competence in practice. Prognosis is perhaps an unusual concept to employ in relation to assessment but since one of the major aims of professional education is to prepare the student to enter professional practice, prediction of the likelihood of the student's competence in it during the early stages of professional practice appears to be a logical expectation from assessment.

Continuous assessment is the most likely form of assessment to offer the basis for any form of prognosis. Hence, it is suggested here that assessment is about diagnosis and prognosis, and the teacher practitioner must necessarily be involved in both.

V Peer and Self Assessment

It was noted earlier in this chapter that most of the forms of assessment discussed were teacher centred but in recent years there have been some objections raised to this approach. Heron (1981), for instance, suggests that teacher-centred assessment is authoritarian, but it is maintained here that although the teacher practitioner has authority to assess, that such authority must lie in her professionalism rather than her delegated authority as a teacher practitioner, so that teacher-centred assessment is important in professional education. Nevertheless, it is also recognised that the teacher practitioner also has authority delegated from the profession to conduct an assessment, and that the two types of authority are different. However, there is a sense in which teacher centred assessment is incongruous, if the teacher practitioner and the student have practised collaboration throughout the period of that practice. Therefore, it is necessary to focus upon two learner-centred approaches to assessment, peer and self assessment. The latter is clearly significant in any form of collaborative assessment but before this is discussed the former is examined.

Peer Assessment: This is a form of assessment in which peers, in this case learners, assess each other. It is a useful method when it is possible to have at least two students working together, which a teacher practitioner may have in the hospital situation but which may be less likely in the community. Nevertheless, even in the community it is possible for students to visit each other and to work together occasionally. In these instances, one learner may observe another and then discuss with her the points that she observed. Obviously this may be seen both as an extension of formative assessment but also of discussion methods in teaching and learning. A frequent criticism of this approach is that students are not experts and so this is a case of 'the blind leading the blind'. There is research that suggests that students may be more realistic in their expectations of their peers than they are of their own work (Rowntree 1977:146), but this finding does not obviate the usefulness of this approach, since the teacher practitioner may also learn what students observe and what they miss in their observations. If this technique is employed it may also be useful for the teacher practitioner to know something about the dynamics of the whole learner group beforehand because some students may also be influenced by their relationships with each other, as well as the performance that they observe.

Self Assessment: Self assessment is precisely what it says it is: that the learner should be encouraged to undertake an appraisal of her own work and then, perhaps, to discuss her assessment with the teacher practitioner. Frequently, self assessment is employed in programmed learning techniques in education where the objectives have been clearly set and the student can assess her own progress. However, it has been consistently maintained in this text that in professional practice the collaborative enterprise between teacher practitioner and learner depends upon there being a continuing process of self assessment by the student. Rowntree (1977:146) reports that when students are asked to self assess and grade written work there is evidence that some students try to guess the grade that the tutor would have assigned while others are over-generous. Clearly the teacher practitioner may find a learner who attempts initially to say what she thinks that the teacher practitioner wants her to say about her practice but, in this instance, it is the responsibility of the teacher practitioner to probe more deeply and to discover what the learner really thinks. After a period of working together a more open relationship should be created in which the problem does not arise. Over-generous rating of a performance, however, is useful in diagnostic appraisal since it enables the teacher practitioner to become aware of the standards, knowledge and expectations of the student. Thus the teacher practitioner is in a position to discuss these with the student, where appropriate.

However, this suggests that self assessment is only used in a teacher based manner and this would be a false idea. By listening to the student the teacher practitioner should learn a great deal about what she considers her needs to be and since adult students learn best when they see the relevance of what they are doing it is important that the teacher practitioner responds to the expressed learning needs of the student. Self assessment is, therefore, quite crucial to the whole process of teaching and learning in an individualised, non-formal manner. Hence the teacher practitioner should, from the outset, encourage this approach; be prepared to listen to what the student says, adopt a socratic approach to assessment after a role performance and continually encourage the student to reflect upon what she has done in order to facilitate the learning process. However, it is suggested here that self assessment during the professional practice experience should not be isolated from professional practice after qualification, so that the teacher practitioner has a further role in this respect.

VI Teaching the Art of Self Assessment

A professional practitioner is one who endeavours to be the master of the discipline upon which her practice is based so that she can render the best possible service to her clients. However, the professional's practice is ultimately the basis upon which her clients and maybe her colleagues will judge her, so that in order to provide that excellent service she has to be a good practitioner as well as a good theoretician. Hence, her practice, the implementation of procedures/skills and the way that she interacts with clients and colleagues, is fundamental to her professionalism. Therefore the professional needs constantly to be able to assess herself because once she is a fully fledged professional she is unlikely to be assessed very frequently by others in such a manner as to benefit her own practice.

It is, therefore, maintained here that the art of self assessment should be taught to all intending professional practitioners during their preparation and for nurses, midwives and health visitors this is one of the elements of the role of the teacher practitioner. Not only does she encourage the student to self assess her own learning needs but she must help the student assess her practice, so that she will develop the habit of assessing this when she has qualified. This habit will not be developed if the teacher practitioner makes her comments on the role performance before listening to the student's. Moreover, the teacher practitioner, through shrewd questioning, might actually help the student to gain more insight into her own practice. In the first instance, the teacher practitioner may help the student undertake this when she has been present and witnessed the role performance but as the period of professional experience proceeds she might well wish to help the student assess her practice without actually being present at the role performance. A number of techniques are useful in this instance:

- a socratic tutorial, in which the teacher practitioner asks the student about the role performance and continues to raise questions in order to assess it

- a prepared checklist of questions, so that the student is expected to work through the questions after a role performance in order to get into the habit of analysing the process

- a written record and assessment of each role performance for the teacher practitioner to read. In this way the student is expected to write an assessment, but if that is regarded as only being for the teacher practitioner's benefit, it may not help the student sufficiently to develop the habit of self assessment.

It will be recalled that the learning cycle, discussed earlier in this book, has a stage of reflectivity and it is at this point that the teacher practitioner must encourage the student to reflect upon her practice and to learn from it, so that she is always endeavouring to improve her practice for the benefit of her clients/patients.

Conclusion

The teacher practitioner is, therefore, both the assessor and the teacher of assessment technique to encourage the student to develop the habit of self-assessment but the teacher practitioner must also be totally professional herself so that her professional practice, as teacher and practitioner, should also be open to her own self-appraisal. Yet there is a sense in which she is fortunate because, provided that she has developed a good relationship with the student with whom she is working she has a colleague who is able to comment upon her professional practice and help her to continue to improve the service she offers to patients/clients and to students. Since the teacher practitioner has the opportunity to help the student, she should also be prepared to let the student help her improve and develop as part of the normal human interaction. The student will assess her teacher practitioner in any case, since this is natural in social interaction, so that the teacher practitioner may benefit considerably by encouraging the student to articulate her comments.

Thus far this text has concentrated quite specifically upon the teaching role of the teacher practitioner, but the next chapter widens the focus and examines the whole process of which the teacher practitioner is but one part.

Chapter Seven

PERSPECTIVES ON THE EDUCATIONAL PROCESS

The previous chapters of this book have focused upon the teaching and learning process but it is now necessary to locate this within a much wider context, so that the teacher practitioner may see her role against the broader backcloth of nursing, midwifery and health visiting. In addition, this chapter will introduce some of the theoretical issues that underlie the discussion contained in the previous ones, so that the latter two parts are necessarily more abstract. The chapter itself contains three sections only: the first examines the process of implementing a course for professional preparation and the other two discuss some of the philosophical and sociological issues that arise from the actual process of preparing new recruits to a profession.

I The Implementation of a Course for Professional Preparation

Schools of nursing and midwifery and institutions of further and higher education engaged in basic and post-basic education and training of nurses, midwives and health visitors do not act independently of the wider profession. Indeed, the United Kingdom Central Council and the four National Boards for Nursing, Midwifery and Health Visiting have overall responsibility for the preparation of new practitioners. The former is responsible for: maintaining the professional register; establishing standards of professional conduct and removing from the register the names of any who are found guilty of serious professional misconduct; making statutory rules governing entry to training and criteria for registration; improving the standards of training in collaboration with the Boards. The latter are responsible, within their national boundaries, for: approving training institutions; validating courses developed by these institutions from their outline curricula and syllabi; monitoring courses; controlling examinations; investigating cases of alleged misconduct. Each Board has education officers who are professionally available to provide advice when courses are being developed and submissions are being prepared. Naturally, they are also available to be of assistance when courses are actually running. Since each National Board differs in its committee structure and precise mode of operation and, in addition, some of their functions are delegated to the District Nursing and Health Visiting Joint

Committees of the United Kingdom Central Council and the National Boards, a general rather than a specific description of the process of validation is presented here.

Currently there are a number of procedures in operation for the purposes of gaining approval for courses, although two appear to be used most frequently. However, as they are in the process of revision by the statutory bodies, and it is anticipated that details might change, only the broad outlines of these approaches are given here.

The first procedure entails the professional education officers visiting the training institution, having first received relevant information from service and academic staff. The visit may last for several days, depending upon the number of courses under consideration. During the institutional visit the education officers prepare a detailed report about the visitation that is then submitted to the appropriate committee of the relevant statutory body. After consideration, a report is prepared for the training institution and for the District Health Authority which grants permission, asks for changes, etc. This approach is usually adopted for basic nursing and midwifery training.

In contrast, the second approach is one in which the educational establishment prepares a detailed submission which is to be made to the statutory body. This submission is frequently prepared by a curriculum planning group or a course team. The appropriate committee of the statutory body considers the submission and either asks for revision or more information or arranges for some of its representatives (and occasionally non-members) to visit the institution. In the former instance, on receipt of the appropriate information or curriculum revision, a visit is then arranged. In most cases the visiting party will include an appropriate professional officer and the length of the visit will depend upon the number of courses. The visiting party are expected to ensure that there are sufficient facilities and resources available, that the staff are competent to teach the course that has been submitted and that they have prepared for the major eventualities of implementing the proposed course(s). The visiting party may recommend additional revisions, require specific resources, etc. prior to approval. Finally, when approval is recommended, it is usually for a limited period of three or five years. Thereafter a resubmission has to be undertaken. Since most of the teaching centres which submit courses for validation actually have a team of staff preparing their submissions, it may be seen that validation is a time-consuming process but it is undertaken in order to ensure that the standards of professional preparation are maintained at a high level.

Once permission has been given for a teaching centre to proceed to mount a course, the course team have to liaise with appropriate personnel who will assist in the course, such as teacher practitioners, visiting specialist teachers, ensure that the resources are available, prepare a timetable, advertise the course etc.

Not only do all these procedures have to be implemented, but it is necessary to prepare thoroughly the assessment procedures. Arrangements have to be made to conduct the examination and where the responsibility for the assessment procedure rests with the local teaching centre, external examiners have to be approached, approval for their appointment has to be gained and a Board of Examiners has to be constituted. Such a board should include at least one teacher practitioner and a nurse manager, but in the case of potential failure of a student the teacher practitioner who has worked with her might be called to the Examiner's Meeting whether, or not, she is actually a member.

This is but a very brief overview of some of the many organisational and administrative aspects that have to occur before a course may actually be mounted. From this summary, it is evident that any course of reasonable size will require a great deal of administration. Hence, in order to ensure that the course is successful, there should be a team approach in which teachers, teacher practitioners, administrators and secretaries participate. Thus it may be seen that for the actual preparation of the new recruit to be successful requires considerable effort from a team of people and failure by any one member will impoverish the provision made by everyone.

II Philosophical Perspectives on the Educational Process

Few philosophical studies of professional education have yet been published (see Jarvis 1983a), but this section will consider some of the major philosophical issues that have been apparent in this study, which include: human relationships and the authority of the teacher practitioner; the morality of professionalism; the aims of professional education and the problem of indoctrination; the extent to which the preparation of recruits to the professions is education. In addition, the values implicit throughout this text will be discussed in the concluding paragraphs.

Human Relationships and Authority: It was maintained, at the outset, that in the individualised teaching and learning transaction it is vitally important that a harmonious relationship is established between the teacher practitioner and the student. Such a relationship cannot be established if the teacher practitioner seeks to exercise authority over the learner, an authority that may be based upon her differential position within the nursing hierarchy. That position, which gives her certain responsibilities and for which certain privileges and rewards are forthcoming, may be based upon nothing other than her length of occupational service, or it may be based upon her ability, qualification and experience. Such differentiation of roles and responsibilities is necessary in contemporary society in order for it to function effectively, although too much differentiation in rewards may open itself to questions of morality. It has to be recognised however, that all people are created equal in respect of their humanity, even if they have neither equal abilities nor advantages, and in the individualised teaching and learning situation a relationship is not established by exercise of hierarchical position nor manifestation of unequal abilities but, rather, it is established upon the humanity of the participants. In this relationship two human beings bring together their own humanity and their experiences: it is a relationship of equal adult human beings, with the self of each being of infinite value which is to be treasured and nurtured within the social intercourse. Anything occurring within that relationship that threatens the dignity of either participant or the development of the other's self may be considered immoral. Therefore, it is imperative that the participants respect each other's humanity.

What then of the authority of the teacher practitioner? Authority is not intrinsic to the person, it is either attributed because of position or because of the knowledge or skill that a person possesses and gives to others. The former authority is dependent totally upon the relationship between the individual and the organisation in which she serves, it is ascribed without necessarily having been earned, so that while the office holder may have her authority obeyed she may not necessarily command respect. But in the latter instance, the person has earned this authority and is respected for what she knows and for what she can do; this is not the kind of authority that can be written down and institutionalised but it is the authority of the professional. It is the type of authority that the teacher practitioner may be ascribed, if she has earned it - there is none other of value in the teaching and learning transaction.

Professionalism: Throughout the text professionalism has been viewed as an ideology of endeavouring to be the master of the discipline in order to render service of the highest kind to the client/patient. Such mastery is not for the purpose of self-aggrandizement but in order to be of service. Failure to be the master means that ultimately the practitioner does not really care sufficiently for those who are being served to undertake the hard work, the continuing learning, necessary to remain a master. Hence she ceases to be professional, because she does not care sufficiently to give the best service to her fellow human beings and so, therefore, she fails to respect their humanity.

The morality of professionalism rests, then, upon the motivation to provide a quality service and it is this that the teacher practitioner should both exhibit herself and also seek to ensure that those whom she teaches also demonstrate. No teacher practitioner can expect her learners to demonstrate professionalism unless she herself manifests it. However, if the learner fails to demonstrate a professional attitude during her preparation it is maintained that this constitutes sufficient reason for the teacher practitioner to recommend some form of deferment when she makes her report to the Board of Examiners; obviously such a decision should not come as a surprise to the student since the teacher practitioner should have discussed the problem with the student and tried to help her to overcome it prior to making such a recommendation.

The Aims of Professional Education: It is claimed that among the aims of preparing recruits for nursing, midwifery and health visiting there is one specifying that not only should new entrants to the profession have the knowledge and skills to provide an excellent service but that they should have sufficient commitment to render this. However, it might be argued that the profession is seeking to indoctrinate recruits into its ideology. But if sufficient commitment to providing a service is not an aim, then all the claims that the profession makes to provide a service appear to be mere words. Hence, it should be an aim! But does this necessarily make it a process of indoctrination? Is it necessarily a process of inculcating acceptable attitudes into the new recruit? If the intention were to produce new entrants who believe every tenet of an occupational ideology of service then the accusation of indoctrination by intent would be justified. But there are many ways of rendering a service to patients/clients and there are many unique situations in which it is performed, so that conformity may not be intended - apart from the ideology of caring for all people irrespective of age, gender, colour, creed or race. It should be assumed that people who enter such professional preparation have that ideology but if they do not then their candidature should be rejected because they do not possess such a caring attitude. But should that specific attitude be taught during professional training? Professional preparation is about preparing people to care effectively rather than simply to care. In these instances, the aims of professional education should not be seen to be indoctrinational, especially as another aim, that was discussed earlier in this book, is to develop a critical attitude.

Education and Training: It might be claimed that since a great deal of professional education is about the acquisition of skills and the implementation of procedures that is merely a process of training. But the education versus training debate is rather sterile and it is one that will not be rehearsed here. However, professional preparation is not merely about acquisition of skills although it does involve this. Professional preparation is also about having 'knowledge how', 'knowledge that' and 'knowledge why' as well as about acquiring the psycho-motor skills to practise. Indeed, it is a process that involves the whole person, so that the whole person may be of service to another human being: it is about the growth, development and humanity of that person. Yet if, as Dewey (1916:50) claims 'that the educational process has no end beyond itself', then professional preparation is also about training because it also has the aim of preparing the learner to serve others. Therefore, in this sense, training assumes high moral overtones. If Dewey is wrong, and if professional education does have an end beyond itself, then training refers only to the acquisition of the skills necessary to practise the profession effectively, then it is still significant, since without the skills the knowledge is incomplete and professional practice impossible. In either way, training is important. Professional education cannot occur without training and be a complete preparation of the recruit: it is as essential as education in the preparation and neither should exist without the other.

Throughout this text education is presented as a normative process having one of its most significant ends in the development of the participants, both teachers and learners. It is recognised here that the professional's practice is affected by his personal development and good practice will only occur if the person's moral commitment is to service. Hence, ultimately the basis of value must be with the person. The human person has value in himself/herself because he/she exists - and for no other reason. Activities that enrich the person are, consequently, regarded as worthwhile but those which fail to, or more especially do not seek to, are of questionable morality and should be avoided.

III Sociological Perspectives upon the Educational Process

Like the previous section, this can be but a cursory introduction into a vast topic about which little has thus far been written (but see Dingwall 1977 for his study of health visitors and Jarvis 1985). However, this section seeks to provide an overview to some of the sociological perspectives in the educational process that have been discussed in this text. It must be borne in mind that a part of the process of understanding professional preparation sociologically is to place it in a wider social context than that which has thus far been discussed. This is a vast undertaking and one that will not be attempted in this brief study. However there are five aspects that are discussed here: sociological perspectives; developing a relationship; the functions of professional education; the curriculum; authority and control.

Sociological Perspectives: There are a number of sociological perspectives and they may be classified as either 'macro' or 'micro'. The 'macro' approaches examine the social system as a whole and locate the parts within it and these are known as structural functionalist or structuralist, whereas the 'micro' approaches examine the elements of the social system and are symbolic interactionism, phenomenology and ethnomethodology. These five are now briefly outlined:

- Structural functionalism; assumes that there is consensus in the social system and the function of each institution may be regarded as the contribution that it makes in retaining the cohesion of the whole.

- Structuralism; assumes that in each social system there is a potentiality for conflict and social change but that the system is held together by the exercise of power and coercion.

- Symbolic interactionism; assumes that there is a whole range of social interactions on a smaller scale within the social system and that interaction occurs through individuals emitting and responding to a variety of symbols that are open to be read and interpreted. Hence, interaction is a process of negotiation - an approach adopted in this text quite frequently.

- Phenomenology; starts from the basis that reality is socially constructed and that interaction occurs because there are similarities in each person's stock of knowledge.

- Ethnomethodology; considers the manner in which people undertake interaction and this has given rise to a number of studies of communication. This is perhaps the least well known and least frequently used approach.

These are the five main schools of thought in sociology, but no single sociological perspective is presented here exclusively. Nevertheless, a few points have arisen in this study that encourage a sociological analysis and some of them are discussed in this section, although a sociological study of the teacher practitioner remains to be written.

Developing a Relationship: The significance of the relationship between the teacher practitioner and the student to the maximization of the student's learning was discussed earlier in this study. Interactionism assumes that the persons who are interacting wish to achieve a harmonious relationship, but that the roles that they play are open to negotiation. Hence, each actor will be seeking to act in accordance with the way that he perceives the other expects him to perform, so that they will both be seeking symbolic expressions from the other to guide them. Each will adapt his role in accordance with the symbols that are perceived in order to achieve a norm. Clearly the teacher practitioner may have to take the lead in this process since there are status differences that would prevent many students from so doing. Moreover, the symbols that are manifest are not only those that the actor knows he is giving, eg the spoken words, the smile, but there are other symbols, 'given off' which may be less conscious and less intended but which will also be received by the other person in the relationship and interpreted accordingly. Not only are the two actors giving and receiving symbols about how they should interact with each other, it must also be borne in mind that they come from different backgrounds and bring their own wealth of experiences with them to the interaction. Hence, they each have their own sub-cultural differences and these have to be negotiated, so that there is a sense in which their meeting provides an arena for the negotiation of sub-cultural differences.

Functions of Professional Education: Perhaps the most obvious example of one of the functions of professional education is to be discovered in the procedures for selecting recruits for professional preparation. The candidate must have acquired a certain academic standard before she can be considered for entry and she must then undergo a selection procedure. There may be good reasons why nursing wishes to restrict its entry to those who have acquired a specific number of passes in the General Certificate of Education at Ordinary Level, or other branches of nursing, midwifery and health visiting to require other specific entry qualifications, but there is little empirical evidence to sugget that many of these arbitrary requirements actually relate to the ability to perform the professional role thereafter (Jarvis and Gibson 1981). However, they do serve to prevent some people who have not acquired that standard from entry, even though they may have the potential to become efficient nurses. Every barrier to access creates a 'new poor', so that one of the functions of professional education is to select out those who are considered acceptable to the profession. This selection function continues to operate in a variety of ways throughout the whole career of the nurse but the teacher practitioner plays only a small part in the early stages.

Another obvious function of professional education is that it enables the recruit to acquire sufficient knowledge and those skills and attitudes that the profession has decided are necessary before a recruit may be considered safe to enter practice. While the teaching and learning process may be seen as an overt one in which the tutor and the teacher practitioner play a significant part, there is a concurrent process of professional socialization. During this process the student is more covertly acquiring other attitudes that she recognises as acceptable to the profession. In addition, the student is also acquiring a professional identity, so that she can say, "I am a nurse ..." or "I am a health visitor ..." Simpson (1967) noticed how, during the professional socialization process, the service ethic of student nurses was transformed into a technical interest and the students' use of patients as significant others declined as they sought to acquire technical skills. Thereafter, the nurses began to acquire professional values as they were gradually crossing the divide between non-nurse and nurse and as they became accepted within the professional community. Teacher practitioners may witness some of these changes in the students with whom they work, especially if they work with them throughout the whole of their course.

Therefore, when these students enter nursing they will not disrupt the community of the professional group, so that another function of professional education is to ensure that there is continuity in the profession from one generation to the next, since those who have been trained, educated and socialized are able to assume their place in the profession without causing its structures any undue strain. However, it will be recalled that one of the aims of professional education is to create a sense of critical awareness in the students. If that aim were to be achieved to any great extent, then there is a possibility that critically aware thinkers might prove a disruptive influence to the harmony of the profession, so that there is an inherent dysfunction in professional education.

The Curriculum: Lawton (1973:32) suggests that a 'complete sociology of the curriculum would be concerned with (1) who (2) teaches what (3) to whom, (4) by what means, (5) for what reasons, (6) with what results.' Clearly there is a great deal of research still to be conducted in the sociology of the curriculum in the various branches of nursing, midwifery and health visiting. Since little research has been undertaken into the role of the teacher practitioners there is little evidence about the extent to which they have common characteristics in educational background, career paths, career aspirations, etc. Curriculum knowledge, skills and attitudes are specified in many outline curricula produced by the National Boards, but why was specific knowledge included and other knowledge omitted? Why should some gain acceptability (Marx called it sacred knowledge) while other remains less acceptable (Marx's profane knowledge)? Why should curriculum knowledge of a cognitive nature have higher status than psycho-motor skills (Young 1971)? Lawton's third point refers to those who actually enter nursing, midwifery and health visiting. Do they have characteristics in common with those who enter other semi-professions, such as teaching? Are there trends in entry at the present time, caused by social circumstances, such as more highly qualified young people entering nursing since there are fewer other occupational opportunities open to them elsewhere because of the declining job market? By what means? For what reasons? Teaching methods have been discussed in considerable detail in this text, but why do some teachers prefer teacher-centred methods and other learner-centred approaches? Are there common characteristics between them and teacher practitioners adopting a similar approach? Bourdieu and Passeron (1977) claim that teacher-centred methods are a form of symbolic violence which reflects power and authority in the teacher's position - is this valid for some teacher practitioners? Lawton's final point asks which methods have achieved the most effective results in terms of practising the profession. This is another question that requires considerable research.

These are all questions about the sociology of the curriculum, many of which may remain unanswered but some might be answerable by teacher practitioners themselves undertaking their own research. Teacher practitioners, because of their unique and important position, are in a good position to undertake small scale research in their own areas and this would enrich considerably the body of knowledge that exists about this aspect of professional education.

Authority and Control: There have been a numbr of references to authority and control throughout this text and it is a significant area of interest for some sociologists, since education is clearly an instrument in ensuring the stability of a society, a social system or a profession. Hence, some sociologists have examined and related the educational process to the wider power structures of society but little of this has actually been undertaken in nursing, health visiting or midwifery.

Conclusion

Clearly in a text of this length it is impossible to do justice to the intricacies of the philosophical arguments or to the complexity of the sociological approaches. This chapter has merely attempted to provide an introduction to some of these topics and problems so that teacher practitioners may see their role within a wider context and appreciate some of the other issues involved in professional education. In conclusion, however, it is now necessary to return to the role of the teacher practitioner.

Chapter Eight

CREATING A ROLE

This book commenced with an examination of the roles of the teacher practitioner and ends with a brief consideration of the role of the teacher practitioner; it began with a separation of the two roles of teacher and practitioner and it ends with the recognition that there is one occupational role and that it is a very important role within the context of preparing new recruits to nursing, midwifery and health visiting. Throughout the book the theory and practice of teaching adults has been under consideration, irrespective of whether the teacher practitioner actually practises nursing, midwifery or health visiting, because teaching adults is the common element. Teacher practitioners from the different branches of nursing can be prepared together on the same course because of the nature of this common element. To separate them is to the dis-service of their common role but to unite them is to acknowledge the centrality of their educational role and to enrich their learning experiences.

However, in their own professional disciplines, their roles are difficult and demanding for they are both professional practitioners and professional educators of adults. The separation has been for heuristic purposes only, for in point of fact they are simultaneous and concurrent roles. But because it is a different role from other practitioners there is a certain freedom to create the role that the teacher practitioner chooses. It is one that she has to create herself and it is upon this that the first part of this brief chapter focuses. Thereafter, consideration is given to the evaluation of the role performance and, finally, there is a brief conclusion.

I The Expectations of the Role Set

Traditionally, role performance was viewed as a simple dynamic performance that was linked to a status, so that the teacher practitioner would have been regarded as a status position with an associated role performance. Role performance was thought of as being prescribed by the generally held expectations about the way that it should be performed. To some extent this still obtains since the National Health Service is, and probably has to be, a highly bureaucratic organization. However, Merton (1968:41-5) has argued that a status holder actually performs his role differently as he interacts with the different people in his role set. The implications of this are that if all the members of the role set have certain expectations of the way that the role should be played, it is difficult for the role player to resist the social pressures to conform, but if there is a diversity of attitudes among the role set then there is more freedom for the role player to negotiate the way she performs her role. There is, therefore, more flexibility in the way that the role is performed and, in this, it approximates to the autonomous approach to role performance that many people experience.

However, the education of adults is a young discipline and most people's attitudes to teaching and learning might still be coloured by their own experience in school or in their initial nurse training. Hence, it would not be difficult to envisage a situation in which the expectations that some members of the role set have about the teacher practitioner's role performance do not appear to be in accord with her own. Imagine a situation in which the nurse manager thinks that the learner centred approach allows the student too much latitude; the tutor wishes the teacher practitioner to follow a prescribed syllabus; the student wants the teacher practitioner to be more teacher centred; colleagues feel that the approach needs to be more tightly structured: what should the teacher practitioner do? Clearly constant pressure might force her to conform to a more teacher centred approach. But if that is the case, then cultural reproduction may be perpetuated and the teacher practitioner might still be an instructor rather than a teacher of adults. It is in instances such as this that associations of teacher practitioners are important, since members can provide support for each other in their role performance. Such professional associations of teacher practitioners are important because they can act as a forum for teacher practitioners to teach and learn from each other.

The picture drawn in the previous paragraph may not depict reality at all and, by contrast, the teacher practitioner may gain support from all the members of her role set, so that she does not have to explain and negotiate with each of the members. Even so, it is the teacher practitioner's responsibility to decide how she should play her role, within the prescribed parameters of the Health Service, but since she does work in a team it may always be necessary to explain why she is using the approach that she does. By creating her own role, the teacher practitioner may construct something that is uniquely hers and as such is most satisfying to perform.

II Evaluation of Role Performance

The teacher practitioner should be a professional and, as was discussed in the sixth chapter, she should constantly assess her role performance as she plays it with each member of the role set. Self assessment should make her aware of her own learning needs and her professionalism should drive her on to become a self directed learner. The students who work with her may be the only people who observe her perform her role with all members of the role set and, provided that the relationship that has been established between them is harmonious, their comments may be useful and beneficial to help her continue to evaluate her own role performance. For as long as she assesses and re-assesses that role performance she will remain a professional and once the critical awareness of self assessment disappears then her professionalism is in danger. Continual self evaluation is one of the hallmarks of the professional, leading to more learning and the enthusiasm to learn is one of those attitudes that should be transmitted in the process of professional socialization, so that the best service can be rendered to the patient or client.

Conclusion

This brief book has been written for teacher practitioners in order to introduce them to the discipline of the education of adults. Whatever their professional practice, staff nurse, ward sister, charge nurse, health visitor, midwife, district nurse, etc., their teaching responsibility is something that they share. It is hoped that by using the knowledge, skills and attiudes discussed in this book their own role performance may be enriched and that this will be to the benefit of those students with whom they work and, in part, for whom they work.

SUGGESTED FURTHER READING

The following list of books and journals is suggested for readers who wish to pursue any of the discussion in this book. Naturally, any list is bound to be selective but this has been restricted to about twenty five books and journals so that the reader will feel able to make a reasonable selection.

Books on Education in Nursing, Midwifery and Health Visiting

Allen H O	1982	The Ward Sister: Role and Preparation Bailliere Tindall London
de Tournay R and Thompson M A (eds)	1982	Strategies for Teaching Nursing John Wiley and Son New York
Davis B (ed)	1983	Research into Nurse Education Croom Helm London
Dingwall R	1977	The Social Organization of Health Visitor Training Croom Helm London
Guinee R N	1978	Teaching and Learning in Nursing MacMillan Publishing Co New York
Hinchcliffe S (ed)	1979	Teaching Clinical Nursing Churchill Livingstone Edinburgh
Jarvis P and Gibson S J	1980	The Education and Training of District Nurses SRN/RGN: An Evaluation of the Implementation of the 1976 Curriculum in Surrey University of Surrey

Powell D	1975	Learning to Relate Royal College of Nursing London
Quinn F M	1980	The Principles and Practice of Nurse Education Croom Helm London
Reilly D	1975	Behavioural Objectives in Nursing: Evaluation of Learner Attainment Appleton-Century Croft New York
Robertson M	1980	Clinical Teaching Pitman Medical London

Books on Teaching/Education

Beard R	1970	Teaching and Learning in Higher Education Penguin Harmondsworth
Dewey J	1916	Democracy and Education The Free Press New York
Kelly A V	1977	The Curriculum: Theory and Practice Harper and Row Publishers London
Perrott E	1982	Effective Teaching Longman London
Rowntree D	1977	Assessing Students: How shall we know them? Harper and Row Publishers London
University of London Teaching Methods Unit	1976	Improving Teaching in Higher Education University of London

Journals (British)	Publisher
Journal of Advanced Nursing	Blackwell Scientific Publications Oxford
Nurse Education Today	Churchill Livingstone Edinburgh
Adult Education	National Institute of Adult Continuing Education Leicester
International Journal of Lifelong Education	Taylor and Francis Ltd London
Studies in the Education of Adults	National Institute of Adult Continuing Education Leicester

BIBLIOGRAPHY

Armstrong P F | 1982 | The 'Needs Meeting' Ideology in Liberal Adult Education <u>International Journal of Lifelong Education</u> Vol 1 No 4

Battle S and Salter B | 1981 | <u>Evaluation of the District Nurse Course (SRN/RGN)</u> (2nd Interim Report) University of Surrey

Belbin E and Belbin R M | 1972 | <u>Problems in Adult Retraining</u> Heinemann London

Berger P L and Luckman T | 1967 | <u>The Social Construction of Reality</u> Allen Lane, The Penguin Press London

Bligh D A | 1971 | <u>What's the Use of Lectures?</u> D A and B Bligh, Briar House Exeter

Bloom B S (ed) | 1956 | <u>Taxonomy of Educational Objectives Book 1 Cognitive Domain</u> Longman London

Bourdieu P and Passeron J C | 1977 | <u>Reproduction in Education, Society and Culture</u> Sage Publications Ltd London

Bowles S and Gintis H | 1976 | <u>Schooling in Capitalist America</u> Routledge and Kegan Paul Ltd London

Bradshaw J	1972	The Concept of Social Need in New Society 30 March
Chickering A W and associates	1981	The Modern American College Jossey Bass Inc Publishers San Francisco
Coombes P H and Ahmed M	1974	Attacking Rural Poverty: How Non-Formal Education Can Help Johns Hopkins University Press Baltimore
Cooper C L (ed)	1976	The Theories of Group Processes John Lilley and Sons London
Cross K P	1981	Adults as Learners Josey Bass Publishers San Francisco
Davies I K	1971	The Management of Learning McGraw-Hill Book Company (UK) Ltd London
Davies I K	1976	Objectives in Curriculum Design McGraw-Hill Book Company (UK) Ltd London
Davis B (ed)	1983	Research into Nurse Education Croom Helm London
de Tornyay R and Thompson M A	1982	Strategies for Teaching Nursing John Wiley and Sons New York
Dewey J	1916	Democracy and Education The Free Press MacMillan Publishing Co New York
Dingwall R	1977	The Social Organization of Health Visitor Training Croom Helm London
Dreyfus H L and Dreyfus S E	1981	The Movement for Novice to Expert: What Experience Teaches cited in de Tornyay and Thompson 1982 op cit

Eisner E W	1969	Instructional and Expressive Objectives in Popham et al (1969) op cit
Erikson E H	1965	Childhood and Society Penguin Harmondsworth
Freire P	1972	Pedagogy of the Oppressed Penguin Harmondsworth
Hall C	1973	Who Controls the Nursing Profession? - The Role of the Professional Association (Occasional Paper pp89-92) Nursing Times June 7
Hamilton D	1976	Curriculum Selection Open Books London
Harrow A J	1972	A Taxonomy of the Psychomotor Domain McKay New York
Heron J	1981	Assessment British Postgraduate Medical Federation, University of London and Human Potential Research Project, University of Surrey
Hilgard R E and Atkinson R C	1967 4th ed	Introduction to Psychology Harcourt Brace Jovanovich New York
Hirst P H and Peters R S	1970	The Logic of Education Routledge and Kegan Paul London
Howe M J A (ed)	1977	Adult Learning John Wiley and Sons Chichester
Hoy R and Robbins J	1980	The Profession of Nursing McGraw-Hill Book Company (UK) Ltd London
Illich I	1977	Disabling Professions in Illich et al 1977 op cit

Illich I, Zola I K, McKnight J, Coplan J and Shanken R 1977 *Disabling Professions* Marion Boyars London

Jarvis P 1978 District Nurse Examiners - How Do They Score? in *Nursing Times* (9 March)

Jarvis P 1979 Assessment of Teaching in *Journal of Community Nursing* (April)

Jarvis P 1983a *Professional Education* Croom Helm London

Jarvis P 1983b *Adult and Continuing Education: Theory and Practice* Croom Helm London

Jarvis P 1985 *A Sociology of Adult and Continuing Education* Croom Helm London

Jarvis P and Gibson S 1980 *The Education and Training of District Nurses SRN/RGN An Evaluation of the Implementation of the 1976 Curriculum in Surrey (October 1978 - August 1979)* An Interim Report University of Surrey

Jarvis P and Gibson S 1981 An Investigation into the Validity of Specifying 5 'O' Levels in the General Certificate of Education as an Entry Requirement for the Education and Training of District Nurses in *Journal of Advanced Nursing Studies*, Vol 6

Kelly A V 1977 *The Curriculum Theory and Practice* Harper and Row London

Kerr J F (ed) 1968 *Changing the Curriculum* University of London Press London

Kidd J R 1973, 2nd ed. How Adults Learn. Association Press, Chicago

Knowles M 1980, 2nd ed. The Modern Practice of Adult Education. Association Press, Chicago

Knox A B 1977. Adult Development and Learning. Jossey Bass Publishers Ltd, San Francisco

Kolb D A and Fry R 1975. Towards an Applied Theory of Experiential Learning, in Cooper C L (ed) 1975 op cit

Krathwohl D R, Bloom B S and Masia B B 1964. Taxonomy of Educational Objectives Book 2 Affective Domain. Longman Group Ltd, London

Krech D, Crutchfield R S and and Ballachey E L 1962. Individual in Society. McGraw-Hill Book Company Ltd, New York

La Belle T 1982. Formal, Nonformal and Informal Education: A Holistic Perspective on Lifelong Learning, in International Review of Education Vol 28 No 2

Lawson K H 1975. Philosophical Concepts and Values in Adult Education. University of Nottingham, Department of Adult Education

Lawton D 1973. Social Change, Educational Theory and Curriculum Planning. Hodder and Stoughton, London

Legge D 1974. The Use of the Talk in Adult Classes, in Stephens H and Roderick G 1974 op cit

Lewin K 1952. Group Decision and Social Change, in Swanson et al (eds) 1952 op cit

Lippitt R and White R K 1958 — An Experimental Study of Leadership and Group Life in Maccoby et al
in Maccoby et al (eds) 1958 op cit

Long H B 1983 — Adult Learning
Cambridge Book Co New York

Maccoby E E, Newcomb T M and Hartley E L (eds) 1958 3rd ed — Readings in Social Psychology
Holt New York

Mc Gregor D 1960 — The Human Side of Enterprise
McGraw-Hill New York

Mager R F 1975 — Preparing Instructional Objectives
Fearon Publishers, Inc
Belmont California

Maslow A 1968 2nd ed — Towards a Psychology of Being
D Van Nostrand Co New York

Merton R K 1968 2nd ed — Social Theory and Social Structure
The Free Press New York

Mezirow J 1981 — A Critical Theory of Adult Learning and Education
in Adult Education Vol 32 No 1
Washington

Nicholls A and Nicholls H 1978 — Developing a Curriculum
A Practical Guide
George Allen and Unwin London

Ogier M E 1983 — The Ward Sister as a Teacher Resource Person
in Davis B D (ed) 1983 op cit

Paterson R W K 1979 — Values, Education and the Adult
Routledge and Kegan Paul London

Popham W J, Eisner E W, Sullivan H J and Tyler L L 1969 — Instructional Objectives
Rand McNally Chicago

Reilly D 1975 — Behavioural Objectives in Nursing: Evaluation of Learner Attainment
Appleton-Century-Crofts
New York

Robinson J J and Taylor D	1983	Behavioural Objectives in Training for Adult Education in International Journal of Lifelong Education Vol 2 No 4
Rogers C R	1969	Freedom to Learn Charles E Merrill Publishing Co Columbus, Ohio
Rogers J	1977 ed	Adults Learning Open University Press Milton Keynes
Rowntree D	1977	Assessing Students: How Shall We Know Them? Harper and Row London
Ryle G	1949	The Concept of Mind Hutchinson House London
Schaie K W and Parr J	1981	Intelligence in Chickering A W et al op cit
Simpson E J	1966	The Classification of Educational Objectives Psychomotor Domain University of Illinois Urbana, Illinois
Simpson I H	1967	Patterns of Socialization into Professions: The Case of Student Nurses in Sociological Inquiry No 37 (winter)
Smith M	1977	Adult Learning and Industrial Training in Howe M (ed) 1977 op cit
Spruce J	1983	Assessment of Practical Nursing Skills Unpublished MSc Dissertation University of Surrey
Srinivasan L	1977	Perspectives on Nonformal Adult Learning World Education New York

Stephens M D and Roderick G W	1974	Teaching Techniques in Adult Education David and Charles Newton Abbot
Swanson G E, Newcomb T M and Hartley E L (eds)	1952	Readings in Social Psychology Holt New York
Taba H	1962	Curriculum Development Theory and Practice Harcourt Brace and World New York, Chicago, San Fransisco, Atlanta
Thorndike E L	1928	Adult Learning MacMillan London
Trenaman J	1951	The Length of a Talk Report of an Enquiry into the Optimum Length of and Informative Broadcast Talk for the Adult Student Type of Listener cited from Legge D op cit
Vollmer H M and Mills D L (eds)	1966	Professionalization Prentice-Hall Inc., Englewood Cliffs, N.J.
Wheeler D K	1967	Curriculum Process London: University of London Press
Young M F D (ed)	1971	Knowledge and Control Collier-MacMillan Publishers London
	1982	Rules, Regulations, Notes for Guidance and Syllabuses for Courses English National Board for Nursing, Midwifery and Health Visiting London
	1983	Regulations and Guidelines for District Nurse Education and Training and Related Matters Panel of Assessors for District Nurse Training, London Adopted by ENB September 1983

INDEX

Abilities 27,29,81,84,92
Academic Adviser 18
Accountability 15
Adolescence 45
Adult Development 37
  Learners 28,32,48
  Learning 2,39-52,54
Adulthood 39,44-45,48
Affective Domain 20,25,26,28,
  38,39,42,47-49,66
Ageing 44
Ahmed M 53
Aims 15,23,24-27,32,38,43,64,
  75-76,94,98
  Definition of 24
Analysis 25
Andragogy 36,45
Animator 19
Application 25
Appraisal 28
Apprentice 4,14
Aristotle 54
Armstrong P 33
Assessment 2,10,23,30,37,68,
  77,78-89,92,101
  as Prognosis 85
  Clinical 79,82
  Collaborative 82,86
  Continuous 79,81-82,85
  Descriptive 80
  Formative 33,80,81,82,86
  Judgmental 80
  Peer 78,82,86
  Self 73,78,82,86-88,102
  Summative 81,83
Assessor 10,65,77,84
Assignments 68
Atkinson R C 37
Attitude 3,21,26,27,34,47,49
  61,67,79,80,83,93,94,97,102
  Change 49,70
Audio Cassette 47,72-73
Authoritarian 12,57,58,59,86
Authority 14,15,16,35,86,92-93,
  95,99
Autonomy 44
Awareness 42
  Critical 43,98

Ballachey E L 49
Battle S 4
Behaviour 25,26
Behaviourism 30
Belbin E M 48,50,60,84
Berger P L 55
Bligh D A 70,72
Bloom B 25,26,27
Books 5
Bourdieu P 98
Bowles S 15
Bradshaw J 33

Caring Profession 18,20,47
Charge Nurse see Ward Sister
Chart 72,73
Classroom 13,72
Client 5,6,8,33,61,65,83,93,94
Clinical Nurse Teacher 1,8
  Practice 8,9,13,20-21,26
  Practitioner 1,3,4,5,5-6,18
Cognitive Domain 25,37,39,42,
  47,50
College 3,6,8,10,20,29,69,73,
  74,79,90
Community 1,4,6,15,20,61,73,85
  Nurse 4,47
  Teaching Midwife 13,33
Competence 5,6,81,85,91
Conceptualization 42
Conditioning 39, 40-41
  Classical 40
  Operant 40-41
Conferences 6
'Confidante' 19
Confidence 50,51,67,84
Confidentiality 19
Connectionism 39-40
Consciousness 43,52
  Critical 43,52
Control 34
Coombes P H 53
Counsellor 18
Course Planning Team 95
  Work 18
Cross K P 37,45
Crutchfield R S 49
Curriculum 9,10,18,22-31,90,
  95,98

Curriculum
Content 23,24,29,30,31,34,75, 76
Definition of 22-23
Development 10,23,28-29,30
Hidden 15
Knowledge 9
Negotiated 34
see also negotiation
Theory 22

Davies I 24,35,49,58
Davis B D 54
De Tornyay 60,64,65
Death 20
Democratic 57,58,59
Demonstration 15,20,59,60,61,68
Development 21,95
Dewey J 94
Diagnosis 34,36,37,80,81 84,85, 87
Diagram 73
Dignity 14,51,93
Dingwall R 95
Discovery Method 50,52,60-61
Discussion 13,47,49,63-66,67,70-72,84
Advantages 63
District Nurse 3,32,67
Nursing 80
Joint Committee 90-91
Dreyfus H L 60
Dreyfus S E 60

Educated Man 54
Education 10,12,16,28,33,49,90, 94-95
as Humanistic 12,58
Definition of 12
Initial 12,22
Non Formal 53
of Adults 6,15,20,24,34,52,102
Social Function of 15
Educational Climate 17
Practice 1,6
Preparation 3,7,8,9
Programme 10
Theory 1,6,7
Educator 5,6
Of Adults 34,44,45, 47,101
Eisner E W 25,28
Empathy 67
English National Board 30
Equality 93
Erikson E H
Ethnomethodology 95,96
Evaluation 23,24,26,31,37,49, 65,73,75,77,78,100
Illuminative 30
Self 19,49,102
Examination 79,90,92
Experience 12,15,20,21,28,29, 34,41,43,45,46,51,63,67,69, 80,81,84,92,97
Expert 5,6,7,8,14,60,68,86
Expertise 5
Eye Contact 62,63,71,72,76
Facilitate 7,13,42,66,69,87
see also Facilitative Teaching
Family 3
Feelings 20
Female 2
Fieldwork Teacher 1,3,7,13,15, 33,74
Teaching: Rules, Regulations, Notes for Guidance and Syllabus of Courses 3
First Meeting 17
Freire P 16
Fry R 42
Furniture 13,62,72,76

Gender 2
General Certificate of Education 97
Generalization 42
Gestalt Psychology 39,41
Gibson S 32,97
Giles H 23
Gintis H 15
Goals 24
Greeks 54
Group 12-13,49,69,86
Discussion 72
see also Discussion
Guided Reading 63
Guru 14

Habitualization 55-56,57
Hall C 5
Hamilton 30

Handout 18,72,74
Harrow A J 25,27
Health Centre 13,69
  Education Council 73
  Service 15
  Visiting 3,4,26,43,44,47,50,
  80,90,94,97,99,106
    Joint Committee 90-91
  Visitor 1,3,4,18,20,26,56,67,
  88,90,95,102
Heron J 82,86
Hierarchy 14-15,92
Hilgard E R 37
Hirst P H 33
Hospital 1,4,13,61,73,86
Hoy R 5
Humanity 12,14,51,93,94

Identity 4
Illich I 33
Independence 15,44,45
Individual 15,283
Individual Teaching and
  Learning 1,6,12,13,16-17,18,
  28,31,34,40,48,52,53-77,80,
  82,93
    Definition of 1
Indoctrination 27,49,94
Instruction 31,49
Intelligence 37
  Crystallised 45
  Fluid 45
Interests 33
Internalisation 26,27
Interpersonal Relationships 1,2,
  6,12,14,15-18,19,32,35,36,41,
  61,93
    See also Teacher Learner
    Relationship
Interpersonal Skills Training
  18,61,66

Jarvis P 10,12,15,32,33,34,39,
  45,46,79,92,95,97
Job Satisfaction 8,11
Journals 6

Kelly A V 22
Kerr J F 22
Kidd R 12,13,14,19
Knowledge 5,6,7,8,9-10,14,15,16,
  18,21,29,34,43,45,46,54,55,
  56,57,59,63-64,65,68,69,79,
  80,93,94,96,97,98,102
  Educational 7
  How 10,54-55,94
  Levels of 25
  That 10,54-55,65,94
Knowles M 6,31,32,33,35,44,45
Knox A 46,47
Kolb D A 42
Krathwohl D R 25,26
Krech D 49

La Belle T J 53
Labelling 17,82
Laissez Faire 57,58
Lawson K 33
Lawton D 98
Leadership Styles 57-58
Learner 2,3,4,6,7,8,9,10,11,
  12,13,16-18,20-21,24,25,28,
  30,34,45,46,54,60,63,101
    see also Student
  Role of 35
  Self Concept of 47-48
Learning 1,5,6,12-21,31,38-52,
  58,59,66
  and Teaching 2
  see also Teaching and Learning
  Climate 31,36
  Continuing 93
  Cycle 29,37,41-44,55,88
  Definition of 37
  Environment 8
  see also Situation
  Experience 22,23,31,32,36,
  42,65,66,69,100
  Experiential 30,42
  Independent 73
  Lifelong 37,43,52
  Outcome 23,25,28,30
  Programme 14,21,31-36
  Style 46-47, 76
  Theory 39-46
Lecture 49,61,69-72
  Discussion 71
  Errors of 70-71
Legge D 61,70
Legitimation 15
Leisure 7
Lewin K 49,57,58

Liaison 10
Life Cycle 44-45
Lippit R 57
Listen 18,83,87
London Institute of the City
  and Guilds 730 Course 3
London Transport 84
Long H 31,32
Luckmann T 55,56

McCutcheon S 23
McGregor D 58
Mager R F 25
Male 2
Management Theory 58
Marx K 98
Maslow A 32
Master 4
Memory 43,65
Merton R K 101
Methods of Teaching 23,24,30,
  31,35,53-77,80,98
Mezirow J 42,43
Midwife 1,3,4,18,26,33,56,88,
  90,102
Midwifery 4,26,43,44,47,50,81,
  90,91,94,97,99,100
Mills D L 5
Models 72,74
Module 9,29
Morality 92,93,95
Movement 27
Museum 74

National Boards for Nursing,
  Midwifery and Health Visiting
  90,98
  Health Service 101
Need 22,31,32-33,34,37,68,71,88
  Educational 33
  Learning 22,29,31,34,80,83,
  85,88
  Training 31
  Types of 33
Negotiation 12,25,29,32,34,37,
  75,96,101
Nicholls A 23,24
Nicholls H 23,24
Notes 71
Nurse 1,3,4,18,26,32,33,56,61,
  88,90,97
  Community 44
  Manager 3,4,15,92,101
  Teacher 8,13
Nursing 3,4,6,8,25,43,44,47,
  50,80,81,90,94,97,99,100
  Care 15,10,47

Objective 79
Objectives 23,24-28,30,31,35,
  36,49,50,60,64,75-76
  Behavioural 26,28-29,30,75
  Definition of 24
  Expressive 25,28-30
  Types of 25-29
Observation 42,83,86
Occupation 4,5,6,8,100
Ogier M E 54
Overhead Projector 70

Pace 28,44,50,51,60,61,63
Parr J 44
Passeron J C 98
Paterson R W K 44
Patient 5,7,13,15,20,26,61,65,
  67
  see also Client
Pavlov I 40
Perception 27
Personal Tutor 18
Peters R S 33
Phenomenology 95,96
Philosophy of Life 26
Pleasure 39,40,51
Popham W J 25,28
Practical Work Teacher 1,3,4,
  7,13,15,32,74
  Experience 10,22
  Knowledge 9,10
    Low Status of 9,10
Practice 4,6,7,8,9,10
Problem Solving 16,20,41,42,
  43,56,57,59,73
  Cycle 56
Profession 4,5,6,8,9,10,21,26,
  78,81,90,97,98
Professional 4,5-6,7,33,56,88,
  94,102
  Body 22
  Conduct 90
  Education 1,4,8-11,15,29,33,
  66,93-94,98,99

Functions of 95,97-98
Philosophy of 92-95
Identity 98
Register 90
Preparation 8-11,12,20,22,29, 36,85,88,90-91,94,95,97
Professionalisation 5,6
Professionalism 4,6,7-8,15,19, 26,35,86,87,93,102
Programmed Learning 70,86
Psychomotor Domain 25,27-28,37, 39,42,50

Qualification 92,97
Questioning 28,43,59,63-65,71-72,88
Questionnaire 31
Questions Types of 64-65

Radical Educators 15
Rationality 54
Receiving 26
Reflection 28,42,43,46-47,48,52, 55,56,59,61,65,66,74,78,87,88
Regulations and Guidelines 7
Reilly D 25
Relevance 29,40,51,74,76,80,85, 87
Remuneration 5
Research 4
Resource Centre 73,74
Responding 26
Responsibility
of Learner 13,84
of Teacher 13,29,30,32,36,78, 80,81
Reward 40,51
Robbins J 5
Robinson J J 24
Rogers C 21
Rogers J 13
Role Model 6,10,11,20,60
Performance 7,10,100-1
Play 66-67
Set 100-101
Rowntree D 33,80,87
Ryle G 54,55,57

Salter B 4
Schaie K W 44
School Nurse 1
of Nursing 6,8,10,20,29,69, 73,74,79,90
Self 45,47,51,93
Identity 4
Simpson E J 25
Simpson I H 97
Simulation 66-67
Situation 12,13-14,16-17,24, 41,42,51,56,62,72,73,75,84
Skill 2,3,5,6,7,8,9,10,14,15, 16,18,21,27-28,29,34,40,50, 52,54,56,59,60,61,65,66,67, 68,75,79,80,81,85,87,93,94, 97,102
Skills, Interpersonal 16-18, 66-67
Skinner B F 40
Smith M 50,60
Socialisation 26
Professional 97,102
Sociological Perspectives 95-99
Spruce J 81
Srinivasan L 54
Staff, Canteen 13
College 3
Nurse 102
Standards 7,8,10,11,15,20,27, 30,34,35,81,82,83,84,90,97
Stimulus, Response 39,41
Stress 20,66,81
Structural Functionalism 95-96
Student see Learner
Subject 12
Subjective 79
Supporting 20,21,50,61
Symbolic Interactionism 95-96
Synthesis 25,29

Taba H 23
Talk 61-63,68,70
Taylor D 24
Teach 6
Teacher 4,5-6,9,10,12,13,15, 16,24,28,35,53
as Manager 35,58
Teacher
Learner Relationship 14-16, 19-20,32,33,77,81,87,88,96
of Adults 6
of Skills 54
of Theory 54

Practitioner 1,2,3-11,13,14,
15,26,34,53,97
as Researcher 98
Definition 3
Dual Role of 1,4
Role of 1-2,3-11,18-21,35,
43,46,50,54,57,58,65,78,82,
83,84,88,90,100-2
Status of 10,54
Status of 10,54
Teaching 1,3,4,5-6,7,8,19,12-
21,53-77
Adults 4,6
Aids 35,54,72-74,76
and Learning Session 75-77
Transaction 1,2,11,12-21,
27,35,40,51,58,83,93
Centre 10,80,91
Definition of 59
Didactic 58,68
Facilitative 58,61
Models 59
Non Formal 54.57
Role 4,6,7,8,19-21,22
Skills 2,60
Socratic 59,63-64,68,73,74,
87,88
Styles 54,57-59,76
Thematic Approach 29
Theoretical Knowledge 9,10
High Status of 9,10
Theory 4,8,9,10,18,54,55
and Practice 18,29,43,54-55,
87,100
Therapy 40
Thompson M A 60,64,65
Thorndike E L 39
Time 7,8,17,34,35,69,70,71,72,
74,75,76,77,78
Training 4,9,10,28,94
Trenaman J 61,70
Trips 68-69

United Kingdom Central
Council for Nursing, Midwifery
and Health Visiting 90

Validation 29,90-92
Values 26,27,30,42,49,78,92,
95,97
Visits 68-69
Vollmer H M 5

Wants 33
Ward 4,6,7,8,13,15,20,61,79,
84,85
Manager 8
Sister 1,3,7,8,13,15,102
Wheeler D K 24
White R K 57
Workload 7

Young M F D 10,98

Zechiel A N 23